Persuasion in *Clinical* Practice

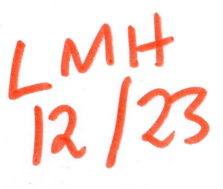

Persuasion in *Clinical* Practice

HELPING PEOPLE MAKE CHANGES

LEWIS WALKER FRCP (GLAS)

General Practitioner, Ardach Health Centre, Buckie
Honorary Senior Clinical Tutor, Aberdeen University

Radcliffe Publishing
Oxford • New York

Radcliffe Publishing Ltd
18 Marcham Road
Abingdon
Oxon OX14 1AA
United Kingdom

www.radcliffe-oxford.com

Electronic catalogue and worldwide online ordering facility.

British Library Cataloguing in Publication Data

A catalogue record for this book is available from the British Library.

ISBN-13: 978 184619 383 5

The paper used for the text pages of this book is FSC certified. FSC (The Forest Stewardship Council) is an international network to promote responsible management of the world's forests.

Mixed Sources
Product group from well-managed forests and other controlled sources
www.fsc.org Cert no. SGS-COC-2482
© 1996 Forest Stewardship Council

FSC

Typeset by Pindar New Zealand, Auckland, New Zealand
Printed and bound by TJI Digital, Padstow, Cornwall, UK

Contents

To Pam, for all your continuing, behind-the-scenes support

About the author

Graduating from Aberdeen University in 1981, Lewis Walker spent the next five years training in hospital general medicine, initially at Glasgow Royal Infirmary where he obtained the MRCP (UK) in 1984, then subsequently at Raigmore Hospital, Inverness. In 1986, he began vocational training for general practice and in 1989 joined what is now a seven-doctor training practice at Ardach Health Centre, Buckie, on the Moray Firth Coast. He was elected Fellow of the Royal College of Physicians of Glasgow in 1998. He is Honorary Senior Clinical Tutor at Aberdeen University and is involved in the teaching of medical students, foundation-year doctors and registrars in general practice.

In the early 1990s, fascinated by what made people 'tick', he developed a keen interest in behavioural change mechanisms, which led him to study both classical and Ericksonian hypnosis, together with neuro-linguistic programming (NLP). To date he has undertaken certified courses at the levels of Practitioner, Master Practitioner, Health Practitioner and Trainer of NLP. With numerous other short courses in addition attesting to his wide experience, he has also trained with many of the leaders and developers in the NLP field. He has the Certificate of Accreditation of the British Society of Medical and Dental Hypnosis (Scotland), and is also a Trainer of Hypnosis. He is the author of *Consulting with NLP: neuro-linguistic programming in the medical consultation* (2002) and *Changing with NLP: a casebook of neuro-linguistic programming in medical practice* (2004), both published by Radcliffe Publishing.

Acknowledgments

There are three people in particular who have made a significant impact over the years on my thinking about how change happens and what we can do to prepare both ourselves and our patients to navigate the process effectively with successful outcomes.

Ian McDermott, Director of Training for International Teaching Seminars, was one of my early trainers when I was finding my feet in what seemed to be a directionless, complicated and often contradictory maze of interventions. Ian brought much clarity to the process, made things simple without being simplistic and modelled an almost effortless low-key style of helping people make significant change easily.

I have been a long-term fan of John Overdurf's material. He is at the cutting edge of investigating the kinds of states that lead to automatically achieving one's goals…and beyond. He has a particular mastery of linguistic applications and I have learned much from listening to and later analysing his specific interventions. One key piece that remains with me is to be always on the lookout for the next smallest step!

Tony Robbins is one of the global change giants who has impacted millions of people worldwide. He has a very energetic, proactive style and taught me that the emotional aspects of change can often be far more important than logical rationalisations. The ability to elicit very powerful positive emotional states and aim them in the right direction can overcome much of the inertia that "stuckness" brings and galvanise focused action for results that count.

I have never met William Miller, Stephen Rollnick, James Prochaska, Martin Seligman, Jim Loehr, Tony Schwartz, Rick Botelho, Barry Duncan, Mark Hubble nor Scott Miller. What they all have in common, however, has been their ability to communicate directly with me through the written word. I have pored over their various outputs, tried it all out first hand, learned from my mistakes and integrated the best of their change processes into my methodologies. I hope that *Persuasion in* Clinical *Practice* may have exactly the same effect on you.

Introduction

What happens when you imagine getting access to *powerful persuasion tools* and being able to *use them automatically* to help your patients (and others, including yourself) get what's really best for their health and future well-being?

This is your opportunity to begin to master influential communication skills.

By the end of this book – *Persuasion in* Clinical *Practice* – you are going to be part of an exclusive group. Very few health professionals get consistently good results across the entire spectrum of presenting problems that are the bread and butter of everyday practice. The skill-sets you are about to learn will help you become one of a select few who can, time and time again, help people make changes in any clinical encounter. I want you to get very good at this – so good that it becomes second nature in every consultation you have from now on.

Before I give you specific details of just what you'll be learning here, I want to ask you a few questions to make sure we are both on the same page. These are powerful questions so I'd like you to *stop for a moment* and really think about your answer to each of them . . .

➤ *What first sparked your interest in persuasion in practice?* With me it was recognising that too few patients really 'followed doctor's orders'. I found that many medical messages literally fell on deaf ears – they just weren't acted on. I began to notice that this was more to do with my failure to understand the process of *how* people made changes rather than their innate 'resistance'. I wanted to be more effective in my work so I decided to learn the kinds of communication skills that could help me ethically influence people in a way that got them what they really wanted deep down – better health. How about you?

➤ *What happens when you imagine getting more of the kinds of results you and your patients want, no matter what the situation?* When I first began to explore this area I was amazed that, even with just a few additional skills, my abilities to effectively reach even the so-called 'recalcitrant no-hopers' improved exponentially. And I found that rather than being 'resistant' to change, many were simply frightened of change. Some had tried and failed and didn't want to try and fail again. Others merely had an emotional kneejerk reaction of 'Nobody tells me what to do . . . period!' And a few just loved an intellectual debate they could win hands down. When I found a few effective ways to respectfully 'get behind the scenes' I found many actually did want help in changing. What if you could get the same results in a short timeframe?

➤ *What is it that motivates you to take action to continue developing your consulting skills?* Many health professionals have a deep-down, genuine desire to help others – that's why they're in the 'business'. Allied to that may be a passion for acquiring cutting-edge tools that can help spread their influence more widely. I am personally fascinated by anything to do with persuasion, change and communication and how I can use that successfully in consultations. What really inspires you in your day-to-day work to have genuine impact on the patients who need help changing?

➤ *What have been some of your most influential consultations for change in your career so far?* For me, it was seeing and hearing the kinds of conversational 'magic' that unlocked the types of stuck states that had kept patients mired in various problems up until now, who then went on to make a lasting difference in their lives. I'm sure you can remember specific consultations, a particular person, where *what* you said, and the *way* you said it, really helped them make a significant change that you both felt really good about. It's a great feeling, isn't it? Perhaps you're not certain just how you managed to bring that about – maybe it even seemed like chance. What would it be like if you could systematically use patterns of effective influence to significantly increase your change consultations, success, giving you even more of that great feeling?

➤ *Are you willing to take just enough control of your personal development in order to learn the kinds of influencing and persuasion skills that will allow you to have an increasingly positive impact on the people you care for?*

Before you answer 'Yes' to that last question there is one thing I want to make absolutely clear. The skills you are shortly going to learn are *not* about forcing, coercing or manipulating people to do things against their will. It is not about making patients do something that they don't really want to do. It is most certainly not about getting your consultation outcomes met at the expense of theirs. These kinds of tactics are not only unethical; they rarely work for any length of time. And, they often leave people feeling battered, bruised, abused and very wary, even untrusting, of any future health messages you offer.

The skills in *Persuasion in* Clinical *Practice* are all about using your influence ethically. They are geared to getting behind the kinds of roadblocks that often stand in the way of effective communication for change. They are about finding out, often on a deep level, what it is that is really important to this unique person, here and now. They will help you help your patients get clear about *what* they really want, and *why* they want it. They will aid you in finding the obstacles that get in their way, resolve any internal conflicts, create an effective plan of action and deal with any relapses along the way. The best kinds of persuasion and influence are the ones that persuade and influence people to do what it is that they really wanted to do all along but perhaps had little idea of what that was or how to get there themselves. It is a cooperative venture where both parties win.

If you can now nod your head and say 'yes' to all that, then read on . . .

THE SKILLS YOU'LL BE LEARNING

Persuasion in Clinical *Practice* is jam-packed full of many, many skills, approaches, new behaviours, knowledge, attitudes and understanding; in fact, everything you need to be fully competent in helping people make changes – whether or not they clearly know what they want instead of their current situation. Here are just some of the things you're going to learn how to use. And when you look back at this list in a few months' time it will be with a growing sense of mastery at how you've been increasingly putting it into practice from day one.

➤ *The five key presuppositions of language,* and how they structure our inner and outer world of experience for both good and ill
➤ *The four common features of all change modalities,* and how paying attention to amplifying patients' strengths is vitally important for change
➤ How to decide which of the *five stages of change* your patient is currently at, and how to nudge them to the next level
➤ *The four principles of motivational interviewing,* and how to incorporate them into each consultation
➤ *Using positive psychology* to enhance the kinds of emotional states most helpful for change
➤ *The five things always present in a problem structure and the five keys to structuring solutions* – you miss these out at your peril
➤ *The seven awareness-raising questions* that keep you on track to get at the real underlying issue
➤ *Going where the problem isn't* – seven questions that help you identify *solution spaces*
➤ How to use *scaling questions* effectively to identify *importance, confidence and readiness for change*
➤ How to become *'response-able'* – being able to respond differently to old problem cues

➤ *The four types of precontemplators,* and how to tailor your questions to each one to encourage movement to the next stage

➤ How to *create ambivalence* in the *raising awareness stage* – often one of the main ways to encourage the change process is to create a problem to move away from

➤ Four types of questions for exploring the *pros and cons of changing and not changing* – it's really important to cover all four bases adequately, otherwise solutions are likely to be both premature and ultimately unsuccessful

➤ How to use *laddering questions* to connect people to what's really important to them –and how important you think that might be

➤ When to use a *decisional balance sheet* plus *'dear diary'* strategies, resolving ambivalence to pave the way for congruent action steps

➤ When to use the *3Rs model,* identifying *results, reasons and right actions,* vital for specifying the details of a solution-focused outcome

➤ *Generating commitment* is a major focus of any change process – use some or all of these eight great questions to generate a powerful state for taking action

➤ *Dealing with obstacles* – why, counterintuitive as it may seem, asking for the biggest obstacle that stands in the way of change can be very productive

➤ How to use four *achievement questions* to unearth past resources and eight questions to identify and utilise *signature strengths* and put them to work

➤ How *energy and state* are connected and how to change them rapidly by using *pattern interrupts, instant state changers* and *changing focus*

➤ How to cue the *relaxation response,* not only as a time out but also as a useful precursor to visualising specific goals

➤ What gets measured gets done, so utilising simple *task sheets* can enhance commitment to making change happen

➤ At follow-up consultations use the six *success story questions* to maintain commitment and stay on track

➤ Prepare for catastrophes by having a *dire emergency card*

➤ *Lapses and relapses* are actually a sign of success – prescribing a lapse can actually prevent one! Should a relapse occur, ask any or all of the nine *learning from relapse questions*

➤ *The* four *major roadblocks* that get in the way of your facilitating effective change – and how to use three *respectful listening* and five *reflective listening* skills to pre-empt this

➤ How to deal intelligently with *negative emotions* that can arise during any consultation

➤ How to use the three *consulting perspectives* and the *relationship process* to sort out challenging people

➤ Several ways to use *'but', 'and'* and *'try'* in a more effective manner – but you don't have to try if you don't want to . . . and . . .

➤ *Persuasive phrases* – seven categories of linguistic interventions with multiple examples, together with . . .
➤ *Changing frames* – 14 different ways to verbally reframe a challenging situation

Whilst this may seem like an exhaustive list you will find many more subtleties and nuances as you read on. Fear not though. The various skill-sets have been sequenced in such a way that you will actually find it very easy to incorporate them into your day-to-day consulting behaviour. And you may find yourself pleasantly surprised just how they naturally show up in the right place at the right time, almost without a second thought.

WHAT CONDITIONS CAN YOU USE THIS MATERIAL FOR?

Well, the real answer is that these skills are useful for just about anything that comes through the consulting-room door. Currently in the UK it seems like we are heading for an obesity epidemic with the attendant knock-on effects of metabolic syndrome, diabetes, hypertension, cardiovascular disease and renal problems. In Scotland the death rate from alcohol-induced liver disease is increasing faster than anywhere in Europe. Binge drinking, unsafe sex, unplanned pregnancy, stress-related disorders and depression are all part of everyday clinical practice. With chronic disease management clinics we have more and more patients on multiple drug regimes to control hypertension, ischaemic heart disease, diabetes, heart failure and chronic lung disease. And of course this raises major issues with medication compliance. We are exhorted (and exhausted?) by government to help people change their lifestyles by taking more exercise, stopping smoking, losing weight and drinking responsibly.

I don't know about you but I see many patients who, without a specific diagnosis, are generally unhappy with their lot in life, apparently poorly motivated to make changes and perhaps even languishing on chronic sick lists without a job or the prospects to get one. Where much psychosocial and emotional distress is medicalised in some way as a 'ticket of admission', we may need to help people not only come to terms with their predicaments but also develop the kinds of skills that increase their internal locus of control sufficiently to learn new coping strategies and behaviours.

At one end of the spectrum may be patients with multiple diagnoses and treatments where we are attempting to juggle medications and pathologies to help them get the best out of life and, at the other, some with medically unexplained symptoms who are keen to seek yet another medical opinion or the newest scan in search of some personally meaningful information to end their diagnostic search. Both groups can present different yet equally challenging face-to-face consultations with no 'one step and you're free', right answer in sight.

Then there are the people with whom we are just plain stuck! They are the ones who come back time and time again and we know just who they are because we get that particular heart-sink feeling when our eyes alight on their names on our consultation lists. These interactions may well be doomed to failure before we even start. It is sometimes quite challenging for us as practitioners to change our perspectives and do something different, mired as we are as if in a swamp with no seeming way out.

One of the reasons I have written *Persuasion in* Clinical *Practice* is because, having been in the same situations with the same feelings of overwhelming responsibility to 'do something, Doc' with many issues not of my own making and with apparent little chance of change, I felt I had to explore any avenue that offered the potential for a different outcome with improved short- and long-term results for all concerned. My patients have been mainly unwitting guinea pigs as I tried out the various skills you'll find in the following pages – and most of them have benefited far more than they could have initially imagined. Here are a few of the presenting issues I've used these skills for:

> ➤ smoking cessation
> ➤ obesity
> ➤ eating disorders
> ➤ substance misuse
> ➤ anxiety
> ➤ somatisation
> ➤ stress-related problems
> ➤ coronary artery disease
> ➤ unsafe sex
> ➤ relationship difficulties
> ➤ childhood behavioural issues
> ➤ sleep disorders
> ➤ difficult patients
> ➤ giving bad news
> ➤ learning disabilities
> ➤ and much more!

> ➤ medication compliance issues
> ➤ lack of exercise
> ➤ alcohol dependency
> ➤ depression
> ➤ obsessive-compulsive disorder
> ➤ sexual disorders
> ➤ chronic illness
> ➤ diabetes
> ➤ other risky behaviours
> ➤ pain syndromes
> ➤ death and dying
> ➤ domestic violence
> ➤ medically unexplained symptoms
> ➤ adolescent crises
> ➤ dementia and memory issues

THE STRUCTURE OF *PERSUASION IN* CLINICAL *PRACTICE*

The first six chapters will give you a firm foundation of the kinds of things that need to be there as prerequisites of any change process. Following on from Chapter 1, an overview of the various validated models incorporated herein together with the 'big picture' of the five-step process integral to each change consultation, we deal with five pivotal platforms.

> ➤ Styles of change – explores each individual's unique way of motivating themselves to do something different and how this shows up in their language.

➤ Problems and solutions – learn to separate process from content. Discover the deeper structure that is always present in any problem or solution, and how to begin to create solution spaces by 'going where the problem isn't'.

➤ Assessing importance, confidence and readiness for change – using scaling questions to assess where they are at right now and begin to increase 'response-ability'. If people aren't ready for change, it won't happen. Yet, skilfully applying this chapter's contents can get people clear on priorities.

➤ Present and curious – how to develop the kinds of consulting flow states that allow you to be present and just curious enough to detect signals of congruence and incongruence which are vital when assessing commitment to change. You need to be able to pay attention to the verbal and non-verbal information that is always there signposting the way.

➤ Avoiding roadblocks – how to avoid the four major roadblocks to effective consulting and develop both respectful and reflective listening skills. Asking open questions for change is essential.

Having built a firm foundation in Chapters 1–6, the last five chapters guide you through the various stages that all people go through when making a change – big or small. You will learn how to assess which stage your patient is currently at, what the stage-specific interventions are, and how to begin to nudge patients to the next level. Each chapter details the kinds of language, thinking styles and mindsets that reflect each stage and gives you many different ways to enter your patient's current 'map of the world' and align your interventions to fit, whilst fully respecting that reality.

➤ Raising awareness – how to recognise the four types of pre-contemplators and begin to sow the seeds for change in those who haven't yet thought about it; creating a problem to move away from as a key way of increasing the initial ambivalence necessary for any change process to succeed.

➤ Resolving ambivalence – having created it in the first place, the job of this stage is to fully explore the pros and cons of changing and *not* changing before coming to a congruent decision to move forward. Using various targeted questions you can cover all the bases and determine what is really important in this person's life.

➤ Preparing to make changes – too many people jump in at the deep end without adequate preparation. This is a key chapter with questions to help you identify results, reasons and right actions whilst simultaneously generating commitment and using signature strengths to overcome any obstacles that may stand in the way.

➤ Taking action – when people are in the midst of any behavioural change they need a set of skills to help them weather the storms that doing something different can bring. This chapter covers various ways of changing state using pattern interrupts, changing focus and relaxing rituals, together with the use of written contracts and tasking to enhance commitment.

➤ Staying on track – lapse and relapse are a normal part of any change process. Key to remaining on track is to prevent a minor lapse becoming a major relapse. Maintaining commitment and having 'dire emergency plans' are paramount. Treating relapse as a context-specific issue can allow you to deal with it as a learning event, resolving any incongruencies and ambivalences that have arisen and generating new action plans.

In between each of these chapters (Chapters 6–11) are five short *Interludes*. Each focuses on a particular set of language skills that can be used at any stage in any consultation. Whilst brief, they provide the kinds of information that can help you deal effectively with difficulties that arise, allowing you to reframe various issues easily whilst paying attention to how you can use language more adroitly for better results.

➤ Kick 'but' . . . without 'try'ing – looks at the everyday words 'but', 'and' and 'try', highlighting how you can use them more effectively to get your message across.

➤ Changing frames – the ability to help someone change their perspective on a problem is invaluable. Here we look at 14 different ways you can use language patterns to transform your patients' outlooks.

➤ Persuasive phrases – this chapter explores seven different categories of linguistic presuppositions so that, before long, you'll just be naturally using them to great effect.

➤ Emotional messages – during any change process, negative emotions such as fear, anger, guilt and shame can surface and derail proceedings. Here we explore the message underlying each emotion and how to use that to create momentum for transformation.

➤ You, me and them – explores the three fundamental positions that are always in play in any relationship. Plus I lay out a very powerful pattern you can utilise to more easily resolve inherent difficulties and challenges.

That, then, is a quick run-through of the key elements you'll be learning in *Persuasion in Clinical Practice*. Whilst the interludes can be read as stand-alone chapters, it's probably best to read the others in order, given that I've carefully sequenced the skills for your rapid acquisition. Before you continue reading on into Chapter 1, you might want to step back for just a moment and imagine the positive effect you'll have on all your patients once you've integrated all these powerful tools and are using them automatically to get what's really best for their health and future well-being. And, with that firmly in mind, I invite you to take your next step and turn the page . . .

Foundations of *Persuasion in* Clinical *Practice*

This book is purposefully light on theory. I have structured it to be both practical and pragmatic . . . using only as much theory as is necessary to support your learning. I want this to be a book which you can easily pick up, quickly access the material you want and begin to use it immediately. The foundations of *Persuasion in* Clinical *Practice* are built very firmly on the *common factors* that apply across all change modalities, the *Stages of Change model*, the skills of *motivational interviewing* and the attributes of *positive psychology*. Before examining each of these in turn we need to say a little about the operating system that underpins them all, and that is *language* itself.

WHAT LANGUAGE PRESUPPOSES

We use language to communicate with each other every day and hardly ever pay conscious attention to the underlying assumptions of each sentence we utter. Yet insidiously and often perniciously, language structures our inner and outer world of experiences for both good and ill. The following principles are the invisible rules that govern persuasive communication.

➤ Language creates realities
  Language does not simply represent the world we live in and experience
  day to day – it plays a major part in its construction and interpretation.
  The very words we use can paint a vivid picture that creates a heaven
  . . . or a hell. Words literally construct something out of nothing. By
  labelling something with a word we subtly create a boundary around that
  'thing', separating it out from its surroundings. Our beliefs, values, ideas,
  problems and concerns are the labels we use to interpret our experience.
  We may think and act on them as concrete realities, yet fail to realise they
  are eminently malleable.
➤ All communication focuses attention

What we say, how we say it, and who actually says it, causes us to pay attention to some things in our field of awareness rather than others. We create foreground out of a background that is made up of everything else we could be experiencing at that time. Language is selective. We can use it directly or indirectly to sow the seeds of change. I might directly say: *'You can learn persuasion skills from this book'.*

More indirectly and perhaps more persuasively: *'I wonder just how easily you'll find yourself learning persuasion skills from this book'.*

➤ We are always influencing

Whatever we say will affect the other person's state of mind and body. Our communication may cause people to move in certain directions . . . even if we say nothing at all. Influence is an inescapable fact of every interaction – for good or ill. Given this inevitability we need to use our language with care so that we can begin to influence with integrity.

➤ All meaning is context-dependent

This is one of the greater insights of postmodernism, especially with respect to language. The meaning of any word or behaviour depends on the frame or context in which it is used. Consider the word *bark*. We can speak about the *bark* of a dog or the *bark* of a tree. The word is the same in both circumstances . . . the meaning, however, is entirely different.

In a similar way we can frame many behaviours – such as overeating, for example – as a problem to be rid of. Or, we can reframe its meaning as one of many possible ways of doing something to make yourself feel good in the moment. What other more healthy ways could get you the same result? This insight opens up the possibility for endless reframes of problem situations, making it a very useful persuasion tool.

➤ Language conveys multiple perspectives

Although we can take many different perspectives on a situation, there are three principal positions from which we speak. These are the personal pronouns of first, second and third position language (I, you/we and he/she/it/they). The interplay of these positions within any act of persuasive communication can be instrumental in creating a problem . . . or a solution. In general, people who are good persuaders recognise the importance of seeing things not only from their own eyes, but also the perspective of their current communication partner and any other third-party interests that might be involved. The information you glean from each viewpoint can allow the emergence of a more ecological change . . . a more tailor-made fit.

Throughout *Persuasion in* Clinical *Practice* you can be on the alert for how the various communication patterns you're learning fit these five basic principles.

COMMON FACTORS ACROSS ALL CHANGE MODALITIES

There are many different approaches to treatment, therapy and change. In fact there seems to be an ever-increasing number of interventional modalities appearing every day – each with its own theoretical underpinnings, rationale and techniques of encounter; each portraying itself to be *the best way* to relieve psychological distress and effect behavioural change; each purporting to be the *numero uno* for a particular patient group. However, research within the last decade (*see*, for example, Hubble, Duncan and Miller, 1999, *The Heart and Soul of Change*) suggests that all approaches are, in the main, equally efficacious. Rather than getting results by the explicit techniques that differentiates them one from the other, it seems that they all share four common factors through which virtually all change is mediated. These common factors (with their suggested percentage effect on the change process shown in brackets) are of vital importance in the process of persuasion.

➤ Patient, person, client (40%)

It seems that it is the personal strengths, resources and skills that the patient brings with them into the session that account for a whopping 40% of the change. These include the person's beliefs and values, how they've coped with and caused change to occur in the past, and how confident they are in their belief that they can change in the future. How they motivate themselves to take action and what supportive factors are present in their home and work environments are also key issues. In short, it is fundamentally important to any persuasion process to highlight and harness these strengths, effectively putting them to work. Failing to do so will dramatically decrease the results you get.

➤ Therapeutic alliance (30%)

No matter what the clinician's theoretical position, all successful change modalities require the presence of factors such as rapport, empathy, acceptance and encouragement. Believing that your patient can actually make the necessary changes is vital. Believing otherwise has been shown to significantly reduce the chances of achieving the stated outcome (self-fulfilling prophecies). Key to all of this is the patient's perception of the degree of support available within your alliance. No matter how supportive you may think you are, it's *their* perception of how well it is functioning that makes the difference. In fact the alliance may well account for seven times the amount of change attributable to specific technique alone.

Together, patient strengths and therapeutic alliance account for the greatest part of a successful intervention. You must pay close attention to both.

➤ Expectancy, hope and placebo (15%)

This effect is due to the patient's belief that this particular kind of intervention is likely to get them the result they want. Everyone entering a process of change has certain ideas about how it may turn out. These ideas can influence the process both positively and negatively. Equally important seems to be the congruency with which the clinician performs the ritual of therapeutic intervention. It is not necessarily the therapeutic model per se but the *belief* that both parties share *about* the model that helps get the result. Bear in mind, though, that this overall effect has seemingly much less impact than the first two factors.

➤ Technique (15%)

These are the specific rituals that make up the particular therapeutic intervention you are utilising to persuade your patients in the direction of their goals. They provide ways of seeing ingrained problems and issues in a new light. Their general aim is really to provide a rationale to prepare and convince patients to take some different actions on their own behalf so that they can alter previously entrenched behavioural patterns. Becoming aware of and utilising many different techniques for persuading change to occur, without 100% allegiance to any one methodology, will give you the flexibility to help many more people.

As I currently see it, the percentage for technique may actually be underestimated. This is because many change methodologies have specific techniques for each of the four areas. There are many techniques to recognise or discover pre-existing patient resources in other contexts, and revivify and bring them usefully into the problem arena to transform it. There are particular strategies that can enhance rapport. Expectancy and hope have a particular structure for each individual that can be elicited and intensified. And of course there are the specific change techniques that each methodology brings to the therapeutic table.

From the foregoing, however, we can see that key to any successful intervention is *identifying and amplifying patient strengths within the context of therapeutic rapport*. Keeping this clearly in mind will help you to stay firmly on track.

STAGES OF CHANGE MODEL

The Stages of Change model as evinced by James Prochaska, John Norcross and Carlo DiClemente (*Changing for Good*, 1994) is a model of how behavioural change naturally takes place in a community setting without the need for professional intervention. Initially researching smokers who had quit mostly without outside help, they found that the process of change seemed to automatically go through various stages. And not only that, they recognised that different therapeutic and change strategies were more suited to certain stages than others. In fact, in applying any specific intervention they found that *timing* was crucial. Each stage demanded a particular approach. Using certain therapeutic strategies too early or in the wrong stage altogether could actually prevent the change from occurring.

The Stages of Change model is a transtheoretical model. It does not promote any one of the 400 or so therapies Prochaska investigated. It simply clarifies the processes of change and fits each intervention accordingly. It frees clinicians up from being blinkered prisoners of their favourite approach and promotes eclecticism and pragmatism. In a sense it is a meta-model of change, which is probably why it pops up with increasing frequency across the varied medical spectrum. In *Persuasion in* Clinical *Practice* it forms the backbone that supports the stage-specific persuasion tools.

In the way that I use the model there are five main areas to consider. We will devote a chapter to each in due course but for now here is an overview of the stages.

➤ Raising awareness

In this stage, often called pre-contemplation, many people are uninformed, underinformed, resistant, avoidant, demoralised, defensive, denying and more. They may not see that they have a problem and may only turn up in your consultation because someone else (a spouse, perhaps) has insisted they come. There are several different types of pre-contemplators – reluctant, rebellious, resigned and rationalising – and we will discuss specific strategies for helping each engage in change in Chapter 7. The main overall strategy in this stage though is to raise awareness about the potential difficulties, dilemmas and predicaments of the current situation. This may actually involve *creating a problem* for them to move away from. Having done so leads them on to the next stage.

➤ Resolving ambivalence

In this stage, often called contemplation, people are likely to be in two minds about what to do. They are now aware that a problem exists yet are undecided, unsure and ambivalent about taking action. In a sense they may want to change and also *not* want to change . . . at the same time. They experience mixed emotions and may feel very stuck, incongruent and often conflicted. They may even go round in circles stewing in the juices of behavioural procrastination. This is a classic approach-avoidance conflict (*see* Chapter 2). The key task in this stage is to explore the pros and cons of changing and *not* changing. Resolution of the ambivalence allows a decision to emerge, leading to the next stage.

Ambivalence is a very important and normal part of any change process. Indeed, without it, change may not occur. So, we actually need to welcome it, promote it and indeed court it in order to resolve it. Remember, too, that ambivalence can also recur during any of the subsequent stages as a signal of incongruence or inner conflict.

➤ Preparing to make changes

With the resolution of ambivalence comes an increasing *commitment* to do something different in the future. If there is no commitment there is no success. Cultivating this state of mind and body is vital. The stage itself is characterised by galvanising and aligning the energies released by resolving the incongruities and conflicts of the previous stage and aiming them in the direction of making something happen. As well as making plans about what *is* going to happen and when (setting specific outcomes), we also need to marshal the various other personal strengths and resources that may be required to overcome obstacles.

➤ Taking action

This stage is all about implementation of the plan and as such requires further commitment of time and energy. It is an outwardly very busy and active period, though of course much change has already occurred in terms of internal thinking style, emotions and self-image. Whilst many people will clear things out of their home and work environment (alcohol, cigarettes, sweets, biscuits etc.) it is also important to know what you are going to do when temptation invariably strikes. Avoiding environmental triggers, substituting healthier behaviours and rewarding yourself for dealing productively with adversity are all part of successfully managing this stage and flowing into the next. Of course, whilst taking action is generally seen as making a specific behavioural change, it applies equally to scheduling a therapeutic intervention for more psychologically focused issues (phobias, anxiety, depression and so on).

➤ Staying on track

This stage is all about consolidating the gains of the previous stages. Behavioural changes are not usually all-or-nothing phenomena – they can wax and wane over time. In particular, times of stress may overwhelm insufficient coping mechanisms, leading to lapse or even relapse. The increasing commitment generated in the previous stages needs to be maintained and further fortified. Because one lapse can trigger a full relapse (and subsequent move back to previous stages) it is very important to plan both for a potential lapse occurring and how you can either avoid it or get through it as a minor blip rather than a catastrophe. There are many strategies that you can successfully use as a clinician during follow-up consultations to keep things on track (*see* Chapter 11).

One characteristic that stands out from the Stages of Change model is the increasing level of *commitment* to change that is generated as each stage progresses. You cannot persuade anyone to do anything on their behalf if they are not committed. More than anything else you need to pay special attention to eliciting, testing for, monitoring and strengthening this state as the *sine qua non* of effective change.

MOTIVATIONAL INTERVIEWING

Motivational interviewing, championed by William Miller and Stephen Rollnick (*see Motivational Interviewing*, 2nd edition, 2002), is a person-centred, directive method for enhancing intrinsic motivation to change. It does this by exploring and resolving the ambivalences and incongruities inherent in the person that up until now have prevented change from occurring. Looked at in another way, it is a method of persuading someone to make a change by using their own individual motivating strategies, beliefs and values in the service of life-enhancing outcomes.

This is *not* a method for getting people to do what they don't want to do. Nor is it about coercing them to do what you want them to do. Unless a change fits with the internal working dynamics of this particular person's psyche and inherent self-interest, it is very unlikely to happen. In essence then, motivational interviewing helps people *persuade themselves* to make changes.

Motivational interviewing originally started life in the trenches of the addictions field. It has now broadened its approach (and appeal) to behaviour change in general. It has spread into many other areas including general medical care, health promotion and social work. There is now burgeoning clinical evidence of its efficacy in helping people make robust changes.

Here are the key principles.

➤ Express empathy

  Reflective listening and the development of empathy and rapport are fundamental characteristics of motivational interviewing. Acceptance of the patient's perspectives, values, beliefs and expectations in a non-judgmental stance is vital. Of course this does not imply agreement with or condoning of these perspectives. Clinicians may differ markedly in their own views and may even express them. However, this is all done within a framework of respect for the patient and the skilful use of reflective listening. The patient's expression of ambivalence about changing (and not changing) is not seen as pathological. It is accepted as a normal and indeed vital part of the change process that manifests in the current 'stuck' feelings.

➤ Develop discrepancy

  At the same time as accepting and respecting the patient's current perspective the clinician also begins to direct their attention through the stuck feelings of ambivalence and on into whatever desired goals, objectives and outcomes they may have for themselves. How does this particular person want things to be different in the future? It becomes clear then that there is a discrepancy between their perception of the current state of affairs and that which they desire.

  The clinician's goal therefore is to develop this discrepancy in the direction of increasing the *importance* of making the change. This is best done by identifying and clarifying the patient's ultimate goals and values with which the current situation and behaviours may well conflict. The leverage thus induced brings about both a change and realignment of perceptions, which become increasingly internally consistent and thus more easily acted upon. In other words, *you are helping patients persuade themselves to change.*

This is of course quite different from coercion, when an attempt is made to persuade another person to change their behaviours because they are discrepant with *your* goals and values (not theirs).

➤ Roll with resistance

Resistance to change is a common phenomenon. The desired goal has both potential pros and cons and requires energy, commitment and movement to attain. When people are ambivalent it is relatively easy to see obstacles looming large on the horizon. Resistance and change are opposite sides of the same coin. Resistance becomes especially prominent when the clinician argues for change and, by a process of psychological reactance, the patient argues against. Deep down inside, none of us really like being told what to do.

Resistance is therefore an interpersonal phenomenon arising within a consultation, and as such the clinician actually has a great degree of control over it. Studies show that being confrontational increases resistance (making change less likely) whilst being more accepting reduces it. You can monitor this by listening out for 'yes but' statements that usually go hand in hand with resistance. It is axiomatic then that the patient themselves make the necessary arguments in support of change.

Resistance = Reasons to stay the same

Motivation = Reasons to change

How do you do this and still keep the momentum for change going? This is where the key skill of reframing or agreeing with a twist comes to the fore (there are many examples in the following pages). This is a form of psychological aikido where instead of opposing the patient's view you align with their energy and redirect it. In this way the resistance to change is displaced whilst ultimately acknowledging that the patient is really the only one who can persuade themselves to make changes. Whenever you sense resistance is present you can use this as a signal that you need to make a different response and come up with a reframe.

➤ Support self-efficacy

Self-efficacy is a construct that relates to a person's belief in their ability to carry out and succeed with a specific task. It is an important motivator for

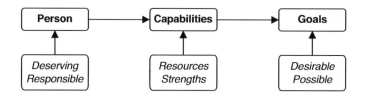

FIGURE 1.1 Determinants of self-efficacy

change. In essence you believe that the desired goal is possible to achieve, you have or can obtain the necessary skills, you deserve to attain the goal and are responsible for taking the required actions (*see* Figure 1.1).

Fundamentally, the clinician supports self-efficacy by using their skill to ensure the patient conceptualises the goal in an achievable format, and identifies, clarifies and amplifies the particular strengths and resources required along the way. At all times the clinician emphasises that the patient is responsible for choosing what to do and carrying out the change. The clinician's role is to help sort out issues of ecology – the consequences of any choice – ensuring that the resultant change is a good fit and match for the patient's personal circumstances.

Very importantly, the clinician's recurrent message is '*I can help you change*'. This of course requires the belief that change is possible for all patients, which has been shown to act powerfully as its own self-fulfilling prophecy.

The key outcome for motivational interviewing is to *get people unstuck*. Creating (if necessary) then resolving the ambivalence that is a normal and natural part of the change process creates a platform on which other persuasion and change methodologies and techniques can be successfully applied.

POSITIVE PSYCHOLOGY

The positive psychology movement is a relatively new field headed up by a renowned researcher on depression and learned helplessness, Martin Seligman (*see Authentic Happiness*, 2003). A turning point for Seligman came when he recognised that, in the main, psychology dealt with problems and pathologies, and that much research in the previous 50 years covered how to explore the depths of problems in order to try to mine for solutions. He saw that the focus was on negative traits and states; as if by understanding how these came about, somehow change could occur. In contra-distinction, very little research was being done on positive emotions (hope, happiness, flow states etc.) and positive character traits (such as inner strength, kindness and integrity).

He contacted several researchers who were currently investigating the psychology of states and traits such as optimism, faith, trust, empathy, courage and valour, flow, love, humour, perseverance, passion, forgiveness, gratitude etc., and founded the Positive Psychology Network which has evolved into its own field (*see* Snyder and Lopez, 2005, *Handbook of Positive Psychology*). Rather than focusing on pathology, the increasing evidence is that by identifying, cultivating and putting to work what Seligman calls *signature strengths* – positive traits that are deeply characteristic of you – we can not only more easily solve our present problems, we can build up our resilience to deal more effectively with whatever life throws at us.

In the 'broaden and build' theory of positive emotions, Seligman's colleague Barbara Fredrickson showed how inducing a positive emotion prior to attempting to solve a problem, learn something new, or even be creative all showed enhanced results over control groups who simply used their habitual strategies. Even a group of clinicians were able to diagnose difficult and challenging cases earlier when their thinking about these cases was first pre-empted by positive feelings.

Negative emotions tend to lead to black-and-white, dichotomous, all-or-nothing thinking, with the limbic system in the mid-brain (our emotional control centre) markedly reducing and even shutting down any cortical input to problem solving (e.g. extreme panic). Positive emotions, on the other hand, appear to enhance cortical functioning and allow far more of our neurology to be available synergistically for creative solutions. It seems that positive emotions may broaden our intellectual, physical and social resources and build effective reserves upon which we can increasingly call.

This fits particularly well with many of the skills of motivational interviewing. For example, Miller and Rollnick are very clear that part of enhancing confidence to facilitate change is in reviewing past successes. In particular they are looking for personal skills and strengths that can be generalised and applied in the current situation. They may even prompt the patient with a list of the characteristics of successful changers and ask them to identify positive characteristics that are stable internal traits.

The message overall then of the positive psychology movement is to focus attention on the development of the particular states and traits that will be of most service in persuading your patients to move from their current situation towards their most highly valued goals. These resources may be different ones for each individual you consult with, yet they will all share the characteristic of helping to develop an internal locus of control that enhances self-efficacy. We will deal with this more specifically in Chapter 9.

AN OVERALL STRATEGY FOR PERSUASION IN *CLINICAL* PRACTICE

In synthesising all the information from these various disciplines we can develop a five-step strategy that you can use in any consultation where the emphasis is on persuading patients to make changes. This will give you an overview of the 'big picture' that you can keep in mind as you consult, whilst successive chapters will go into far more detail about the specifics of each step. In each encounter ask yourself the following questions:

1 *Am I in the optimal state of mind and body?*

How you feel in yourself and what you are currently paying attention to can markedly affect how you consult. There are two principal states that allow you to be both receptive to the nuances of verbal and non-verbal information that patients present and open to seeking alternative solutions that will fit current circumstances. These are the states of being *present* and *curious*. Attending to what is happening in the here and now and developing a sense of curiosity allows us to approach ambiguity, uncertainty and confusion – hallmarks of change consultations – without the pressing need for a quick fix. Tailored, well-fitting solutions are far more likely to emerge instead (*see* Chapter 5).

2 *Have I developed sufficient rapport?*

Therapeutic rapport develops when patients sense that deep down you are allies in the change process, creating a safe space to transform. This results from both avoiding the roadblocks that can get in the way of effective consulting and developing the skills of reflective listening. Without rapport it becomes difficult to identify and act on the verbal and non-verbal cues that abound in each encounter. At worst, from your patient's perspective it can seem like being on the receiving end of coercion. At best it can seem as if solutions simply emerge from the space created. We explore ways to further expand your rapport skills in Chapter 6.

3 *What stage are they at?*

As clinicians we often focus on getting our patients to take action from the outset, forgetting that this is only one of the five main stages of change. Failing to take the time to identify just which stage they're at from the outset will lead to an unfortunate mismatch between their degree of receptivity and the stage-specific tools we are attempting to utilise. This simply increases resistance to change and decreases motivation (both yours and theirs) for the next encounter. Taking the time to get the staging right will dramatically increase your chances of getting successful short- and long-term outcomes. Chapters 7 to 10 explore this in great depth.

4 *How can I nudge them one stage forward?*

We are often guilty of trying to do too much at one time. We sometimes press our patients to take a much bigger step than the one they're ready for. Trying to tackle some problems simultaneously (stop smoking, lose weight and tackle anxiety and depression today!) can be a recipe for disaster. Whilst there is no doubt that some patients can move through several stages in one well-facilitated session, the vast majority need to focus on the *smallest next step* that will allow them to complete the work of this stage and nudge them to the ensuing one. Much change actually occurs *between* consultations. Choosing a particular task as a 'homework' exercise can assist the process, though some people may remain at the same stage for several consultations. You will find that there are many stage-specific tools you can choose from in Chapters 7 to 10.

5   *How can I help them stay on track?*
Staying on track is a judicious mixture of providing a stable platform for change, preventing backsliding, dealing with lapses and relapses and keeping the change process moving in the right direction. Sometimes it can seem like a juggling act. At each consultation it's important to at least mentally review where you're at now and ensure that any previous steps have been consolidated prior to nudging to the next stage. Patients often do slip backwards before regaining momentum and key skills such as reframing and eliciting signature strengths are vital (*see* Interlude 2 and Chapters 9 and 11).

Chapter 1 outline summary

What language presupposes
- Language creates realities
- All communication focuses attention
- We are always influencing
- All meaning is context-dependent
- Language conveys multiple perspectives

Language structures our inner and outer world of experiences

Common factors across all change modalities
- Patient, person, client strengths (40%)
- Therapeutic alliance (30%)
- Hope/expectancy/placebo (15%)
- Technique (15%)

Identify and amplify patient strengths within the context of therapeutic rapport

Stages of change
- Raising awareness
- Resolving ambivalence
- Preparing to make changes

- Taking action
- Staying on track

Ambivalence is a normal part of the change process

Create a problem to move away from

Motivational interviewing

- Express empathy
- Develop discrepancy
- Roll with resistance
- Support self-efficacy

You are helping patients persuade themselves to change

Positive psychology

- Signature strengths – positive traits that are deeply characteristic of you
- Broaden and build – positive emotions enhance cortical functioning

Persuasion in practice questions

- Am I in the optimal state of mind and body for this consultation?
- Have I developed sufficient rapport?
- What stage are they at?
- How can I nudge them one stage forward?
- How can I help them stay on track?

CHAPTER 2

Styles of change

HOW PEOPLE CHANGE

Change is an ongoing process in everyone's life. You only have to review your own history to recognise this. Consider what changes you have made so far in your career. Have you always been in the same position? If not, what caused you to make the change and how did it happen? What about changes in relationships, family and friends? How many times have you moved house – and what precipitated the move? What about your leisure activities, hobbies, sports and other interests? How have they changed over the years? Did you initiate these changes yourself or were they forced upon you?

> *Think of an important change you made in the past – something that made a big difference to your life; something that is personally meaningful and significant. As you read on, notice which factors seem to be particularly pertinent to your style of change.*

Some people like instant change whilst others prefer it to occur more gradually. Instant change is not necessarily done on the spur of the moment, although it can be. It's more to do with having made the decision to make a change, you immediately implement it. Some people do this easily for the small decisions and changes in life (e.g. your breakfast cereal) though some may make monumental, career-defining changes in this way. Instant change can be forced upon you from the outside, however, as in a sudden redundancy or bereavement, and the feelings of loss of control can be very unsettling. More people seem to prefer change to take place gradually, in an incremental way, so that they retain the feeling of being in control. Many changes do take place over a time period and this can allow you to get used to what is happening and customise it more to your needs by utilising ongoing feedback.

Some people like total, huge changes, whilst others prefer them to be partial and smaller in scope. A huge change for some may be deciding to move to another part of the country, or even emigrate. Perhaps you have made a career change into a completely different line of work altogether. Others may view the thought of changing their usual daily newspaper in the same light. Again, most people seem to prefer their changes to be much smaller and partial. Perhaps your change affected only a certain segment of your life, such as taking up a new hobby. For many it is very important that other areas of life are very stable and *not* changing in order to allow them to focus their attention on one specific event. Too many things changing at the same time in various life contexts can be overwhelming.

A change may be quite profound and deep or far more surface and superficial. Profound changes are often about our identity. This kind of change may feel almost like becoming another person. Our various life transitions open us up for this kind of change – getting married or divorced, becoming a parent or grandparent, the death of a spouse etc. Profound changes can be very unsettling when we're in the process of letting go of who we are and have yet to fully become who we want to be. Much change in life tends to be more surface and superficial – such as deciding to buy a new car or change our washing powder. We may change certain behaviours, develop new skills or let go of some old beliefs but we still retain our sense of self, who we are, at a deeper level. Even then, the cumulative effect of many small changes can add up over time and help us gradually evolve almost without noticing.

Some people like to initiate change by starting to do new things, while others prefer to stop doing old behaviours. You may have decided to start an exercise programme to enhance your health and fitness, or decided to stop smoking to get the same benefits. Perhaps you even combined the two approaches. However we look at it, though, all change requires doing something different from our usual, habitual ways.

So, what were your own preferences in making changes? Did you, like most people, prefer that things generally remained the same and only gradually evolved incrementally in a relatively comfortable and stable way over a certain period of time? Or did you prefer your changes to be more radical, completely different from what you'd previously done, perhaps even revolutionary in nature? When you were reading the last few paragraphs you could probably identify with all of the various styles of changing. You likely had other examples from various times and contexts of your life that were a match and fit for each preference. Change happens throughout our personal history in a variety of different ways even though we may have our particular favourites.

Patient change

Change has happened throughout our patients' lives too. In persuading people to make changes that will positively impact on their future, it is vitally important to find out how they have caused change to happen already, in other life circumstances. Making successful changes in the past can serve as a very useful template and resource for making changes here and now. The very skills and attributes they used back then can be dusted off, revitalised and put to work in the current situation. Of course the beauty of reminding people of their strengths in this way is that it further develops their internal locus of control, increases their perceived self-efficacy and gives them a very useful tool of autonomy for making future changes.

It is very important as a clinician to become change-focused to the point of *always* looking and listening out for change-talk and validating it whenever it occurs. Change is part of life and we can be certain that it is always happening. We need to welcome and explore every opportunity to highlight it in our patients' narratives whenever we find it occurring. Change may even have already taken place in the interval between the patient deciding to make an appointment and turning up on your doorstep, so it's always useful to enquire about this.

Here are some questions that can help elucidate change strategies. You don't need to ask them all.

Box 2.1 Change questions

What changes have you already noticed since making your appointment?
How have changes happened for you in the past? (Name various contexts)
What were you doing that helped the change along?
How did you know to do what you did?
What kinds of things were you focusing on?
What did you do when you were stuck to get unstuck?
How did you deal with any difficulties that got in the way?
What did it feel like having successfully made that change?
What is it about you that helped you do all that?
What lessons can you apply to your current situation?

Successful past change in any life context is both an excellent resource and a predictor of future change. You must ensure that one of your very first tasks in any persuasion consultation is to *focus on unearthing your patients' already inherent skills for change.*

MOTIVATION STYLES

How do you motivate yourself to make changes? When you've persuaded yourself in the past to do things that were important for you to achieve, how did you do it? I'm almost certain that you'll have had times when you were really determined to do something . . . and you did it successfully: times when you were absolutely committed to the task in hand and nothing got in your way; times when you've been in a flow state and were completely focused on your goal ahead, to the exclusion of all else. So how did you motivate yourself to get started? What steps did you take? And what would happen if you could help your patients tap more effectively into their own intrinsic motivation for change?

Two styles of motivation

Essentially, people motivate themselves in only two ways: *away from* what they don't want to have happen . . . and *towards* what they do want. Some people use primarily one style whereas others use a mixture of the two.

When people use an *away from* style they tend to focus largely on the problems they want to avoid. They may make vivid internal movies of how bad things are, how much worse it might get and what it might be like to fail miserably with their attempted problem-solving strategies. They may ruminate about what family, friends, work colleagues and various significant others may think if they fall short of the mark. If you have ever waited for a last-minute deadline to galvanise you to do a piece of required work then you have already used this style to motivate yourself. It's a bit like giving yourself a big painful push or prod. The question underlying this style is:

> *What is the worst that can happen . . . and how can I avoid this?*

When people use the *towards* style, on the other hand, they tend to focus largely on solutions – what they want to have happen instead. They may imagine in their mind's eye what it looks and feels like, having successfully accomplished their goal. They focus on the completed task and feel almost magnetically drawn towards it. It's like being pulled effortlessly along. They may even speculate on how family, friends and colleagues may congratulate them on their achievements. The question underlying this style is:

> *What is the best that can happen . . . and how can I make this even better?*

Neither style of motivating yourself is intrinsically better than the other. Both ways work. The *away from* motivation style uses the avoidance of pain to get results. If this is the only way that is utilised over time then the negative internal physiological states it generates can feel very stressful. Sometimes this can lead to overwhelm and a downwards spiral of feeling extremely stuck within a poorly resourceful state. In contradistinction, the *towards* motivation style uses the pulling power of pleasure to get results. It tends to build very positive, healthy states of mind and body.

A general strategy to help people motivate themselves to take action is to utilise both motivation styles. You can simply ask both sets of questions and build up a sensory-rich picture in their mind's eye (what they'll see, hear and feel). Of course sequencing is very important here. You'll want to start with the *away from* questions and pictures first then finish with the *towards* images of success, basking in the great feelings.

Many of our patients are not initially coming to see us about changing. In essence they are using this strategy in reverse to prevent change from happening. They may think of change as being challenging, difficult, uncomfortable and even frightening, and therefore move away from it. The status quo of the current situation then seems safe, secure and inviting even if the longer-term consequences of their behaviours on their health are not. They just can't bring themselves to leave its comfortable pull.

The key intervention in these circumstances is to:

> *Make changing comfortable and safe . . . and make <u>not</u> changing <u>un</u>comfortable and <u>un</u>safe.*

We will explore more of this kind of sequencing of motivation styles in Chapter 8.

Lack of motivation

People who are stuck and have made little or no headway with change processes are often accused –unfairly in my view – of being unmotivated or poorly motivated to change. As clinicians, we often give information and advice about behavioural and other change and when our prescriptions go unheeded we are quick to blame the patient for the ensuing lack of action. In many respects we may be equally responsible for unwittingly helping to maintain the status quo.

> *People are <u>always</u> motivated for something – the question is, what for?*

TYPES OF CONFLICT

When patient and clinician are motivated by different goals, conflict may arise. As we push in one direction they may push back in another. We may want them to change but they may be motivated to stay put. The harder we try to force the issue the more entrenched the situation becomes. In this type of situation motivation can be seen as an interpersonal phenomenon that arises within the consultation. The simple answer to this conundrum is for us to stop pushing our own agenda for change and begin to find out just what this particular patient's internal motivations really are. We need to discover just what it is that they ultimately value, and to see whether their current behaviours, goals and aspirations align . . . or not.

A more intrapersonal stuck state that masquerades as lack of motivation (or even procrastination) is the ubiquitous approach-avoidance conflict. This is akin to saying: *I want to . . . and I don't want to.* In this condition patients may feel very stuck indeed. They want to make changes *and* they don't want to change. The two feelings may be experienced simultaneously or sequentially. A smoker may light up a cigarette and simultaneously experience feelings of pleasure and disgust. A binge eater may derive great pleasure during gorging, then afterwards experience pangs of guilt and remorse (sequential).

Approach-avoidance conflicts happen when we are motivated both *towards and away from* something at the same time. We are both attracted and repulsed by the same thing in a yo-yo effect (cigarettes, food, even a particular person or relationship). If we haven't already accomplished a change we say we really want to have happen – for example, stop smoking, stop bingeing – it is because we have also associated pain to that very same outcome. In other words: *something keeps me hanging on.*

One thing worse than this is the double approach-avoidance conflict. This occurs when there are two choices, both of which have good and bad points (towards and away froms). The closer we move towards one, the less attractive it seems and the more the second option appeals – and vice versa.

For completeness sake there are two other types of conflict to mention. The *towards-towards* (or approach-approach) conflict is when you have a choice between two equally enticing alternatives. Two friends invite you on holiday to different places at the same time, both of which you would love to visit. You win, whichever one you choose. However, beware; people are very good at turning these into double approach-avoidance issues when they contemplate any potential downside of either choice.

An *away from-away from* conflict (avoidance-avoidance) is having a choice between two unattractive alternatives. You are caught between the devil and the deep blue sea. You need to lose weight because none of your clothes fit you and make you look unattractive, but if you do succeed in losing weight you can't afford a new wardrobe. The trick with these kinds of conflicts is to unearth any hidden benefits that both sides could offer.

All of these types of issues and conflicts are best sorted out by assuming they are a form of ambivalence. We will deal with their resolution in Chapter 8.

LANGUAGE AND MOTIVATION FOR CHANGE

Whether or not people are motivated to make changes often shows up in the kind of language they use when discussing what they want to do. For example most people often *don't* do what they say they should, and *do* do what they say they shouldn't. Compare and contrast the following statements and intuit what you think is likely to happen.

> *I really should go to the gym tonight.*

> *I really shouldn't have that last piece of chocolate cake.*

The chances of going to the gym are low and the chances that there will not be any chocolate cake left for anybody else are high. What I suggest you do now is to think of a change that you want to make personally or some task that you have said you will do but have been putting off. As you picture this in your mind's eye right now, notice how the following statements affect your experience.

> I ought to . . . X . . . (where X is your change or task).

> I should . . . X . . .

> I mustn't . . .

> I may not . . .

> I had better . . .

> I wish I could . . .

> I intend to . . .

> I choose to . . .

> I can . . .

> I will . . .

> I'm going to . . .

These are all words of possibility, probability and necessity, both with and without negation (see the appendix for more). Notice which of the statements pulled you towards your goal. Which ones pushed you? Did you push back? Perhaps some had no effect at all, leaving you motionless. Notice which statements made it less likely that you would attempt the task. Did they push you away from your target or pull you away from the comfort of inactivity? Which of the statements made it most likely that you were really going to take action?

People who are proactive about initiating and maintaining change generally use words that imply choice – together with an internal locus of control. They act congruently in alignment with their values. They will say things like: '*I'm going to change because I really want to . . .*' It is uncommon to see these people in clinical practice – they are usually self-initiators of change.

Those who use words such as *ought, should, have to,* are filled with a sense of inner obligation. This is a signal about ambivalence and even internal conflict. It is almost as if they have introjected some parental or other authoritarian dogma (tobacco/alcohol advertising perhaps) with which they have an ongoing debate. This is a clue that both sides of the argument need to be unearthed and heard before a negotiated settlement can take place. These kinds of issues are very common in clinical practice.

Some people may not answer the questions at all. They may have a '*who cares/why bother*' attitude of resigned indifference. This can be a valuable sign of an underlying depression or existential angst reflecting being cast adrift from personal guiding values – what Martin Seligman calls 'learned helplessness'. When people display a seeming lack of motivation and energy for change it is important to address these deeper underlying issues first.

This is of course entirely different from a '*fuck you*' response, which has loads of energy behind it! On the face of it this may seem to indicate a personality or antisocial behaviour disorder. However it is often more useful to put this into the category of polarity responder – someone who doesn't want you tell them what to think or do. This is a major clue (!) about resistance to change and there are many ways to further address this scenario.

Often patients (ourselves included), may initially think that changing their current situation is well nigh impossible. You can use the various phrases above, not only to monitor whereabouts in the change continuum they lie, but also to help them open up to the possibility of changing in the future. Take your own task or personal change issue from above and think about it as you read the following.

> *Some people feel it's not possible to change this . . . perhaps because they think they don't need to . . . or perhaps they can't yet see what to do instead . . . and maybe you shouldn't have to believe that you could . . . change this now I mean . . . You really mustn't think that it's possible to intend to do this easily yet . . . unless you're beginning to believe that you deserve to get what you want . . . don't you?*

You can generate more examples of using language to lead someone from what they consider impossible, bridging the gap towards opening them up to what is possible, by using the lists in the appendix.

Chapter 2 outline summary

Change styles
- Instant/gradual
- Total/partial
- Many at once/one thing at a time
- Deep/superficial
- Initiate new behaviours/stop doing old behaviours

Always ask change-style questions to unearth already inherent skills for change
Make changing comfortable and safe . . .
Make not changing uncomfortable and unsafe

Motivation styles
- *Away from* – What is the worst that can happen . . . and how can I avoid this?
- *Towards* – What is the best that can happen . . . and how can I make this even better?

Lack of motivation
People are <u>always</u> motivated for something; the question is, what for?

Types of conflict
- *Approach/approach* – Towards two attractive outcomes – a dilemma
- *Avoidance/avoidance* – Away from two unattractive outcomes – 'between the devil and the deep blue sea'
- *Approach/avoidance* – Towards and away from one outcome simultaneously or sequentially (the commonest presenting pattern) – 'I want to . . . and I don't want to'
- *Double approach/avoidance* – Towards and away from two different outcomes, both with attractive and unattractive features – the 'grandaddy' of all conflicts

Language and motivation
- *Obligation/necessity* – 'ought', 'should', 'must', 'have to' (plus negation) – implies ambivalence/incongruence/inner conflict
- *Possibility/choice* – 'intend', 'choose', 'can', 'will', 'going to' – implies congruence and alignment with values

Problems and solutions

STRUCTURE AND CONTENT

When people are stuck within a particular problem situation, behaviour or way of thinking there are, at the minimum, two ways to engage with them. The first, and most usual, is at the level of the content of the problem. This is the storyline or current narrative that the patient uses to explain and make some sense out of what is happening to them. It is not 'the truth', merely what they *believe* to be true about the situation and how they represent that to themselves. Yet as you listen to that story, in depth, it is so easy to become seduced into thinking that *that* is where the action really lies.

At times our patients can mimic great hypnotists in their ability to entrance us into believing their helpless, hopeless plight. We can easily get sucked into the emotional roller coaster of highs and lows as their tale unfolds. If we get lost in the content of the storyline then we usually lose track of where the real action is. Not only that, we may find ourselves feeling the same stuck feelings. If you have ever consulted with three depressed patients in a row and become tired, lethargic and frustrated you will know exactly what I mean.

The structure of a problem, in contrast, is the scaffolding or glue that holds it all together. In a sense it is one level removed from the storyline content. It consists of the repetitive thinking, feeling and behavioural *patterns* through which the content flows. Usually, at least until you get familiar with thinking in this way, structures can appear invisible. Yet when you begin to see them more clearly you can use them as a template to help persuade patients to move more easily towards solution structures.

Whereas problems seem to come in all shapes and sizes depending on the narrative, the thinking styles that make up the structure of most problems are remarkably similar across the board. Here are the five categories that make up this structure in its common format.

Problem structure

➤ *Away from* – People identify and continuously focus and ruminate on what's wrong in the situation, on what is *not* wanted, on what they want to move away from. They may do this very intensely and get caught up even more in the negative feelings. They establish avoidant goals such as 'I just don't want to be depressed' or 'I want to stop drinking/overeating/ taking drugs' etc. This saps mental and physical energy leaving little left to actually take action.

➤ *Reactive* – They indulge in wishful thinking. They may consider and analyse the situation over and over again but fail to act. Rumination locks people up in their own minds, stops them being available to other people in relationships and causes them to fail to notice potential solutions in the external world. Some people wait for a miracle to occur. They take little action on their own behalf, often because they say they are waiting for the right moment. They may feel quite resigned and 'tired all the time'.

➤ *External locus of control* – Problems happen *to* them. They may be victims of outside circumstances beyond their apparent control. There's nothing they can do about it, and even if there were, they don't believe they have the necessary skills. They are unable to discriminate what is really in their control from what is not, and fall into a state of Seligman's learned helplessness. Perhaps some kind rescuer will save the day and in one bound they will be free.

➤ *Chunk up* – They take everything wrong that's happening and chunk it all up into a big overwhelming picture. This big picture is bigger than they are; consequently, they feel very small in comparison and even more hopeless as a result. Try this for yourself. Take a small worry, make a picture of it in your mind's eye then really blow it all out of proportion so that it's bearing down on you from a great height and is so vast that there appears to be no way through.

➤ *Options with no procedures* – People with problems are often quite procedural in their thinking and behaving. They do the same things over and over again in a problem context, following the same sets of rules even though they get the same poor result each time. Initially it may seem that they are bereft of any options. When questioned though, they can often come up with several options about what could be done in the problem situation, which initially may seem surprising. They may know that other people in similar situations have succeeded in finding solutions. Why don't they take action then? They simply feel they can't. The problem is that they don't know *how* to put any of these options into effect. They don't know the steps to take and end up feeling even more helpless. And sometimes, in today's fast-moving world of instant information technology, having too many options or choices can lead to overwhelm, resulting in inertia.

For example, let's take a smoker who wishes to stop smoking. They may focus on the pain of stopping (away from). They want to do it but today is not the right time, maybe next week (reactive). When people offer them a cigarette they can't say no (external locus). There are so many hassles right now (kids, spouse, work etc.) that they need a cigarette to relieve the stress of it all (chunk up). They're not sure if any of the current treatments – chewing gum, patches, medication, hypnosis, going 'cold turkey', say – could work for them, and fail to take the necessary steps (options without procedures).

As an exercise it would be useful for you to think about these typical presenting problems in the same format: lack of exercise, obesity, binge eating, alcohol excess, anxiety, depression, poor compliance with medication, risk-taking behaviours, addictions and so on.

Structuring solutions

Whereas there may be myriad ways of solving problems, we are once again at the two-level construct of content and structure. Most solutions share a similar structure regardless of what specific content passes through it. So, rather than having to find a particular solution to a particular patient problem we can ensure that whatever we come up with shares the following solution format.

➤ Towards – Solutions focus specifically on what you really want to have happen instead. A detailed, behaviourally based goal, imagining vividly not only the final outcome and beyond but also the main steps to its achievement is vital. This gives rise to positive emotions and feelings.

➤ Proactive – Proactive thinking helps people initiate action. They stop overanalysing and take the first steps towards their goals. They may not always get things right first time but they use feedback to ensure they are heading in the right direction. They feel energised.

➤ Internal locus of control – Being solutions-focused requires taking responsibility for making the changes you want to have happen. No one can do it for you. Whatever the problem situation, you do have choices about how you respond. All effective problem resolution increases your internal locus of control. Rather than waiting to be rescued, you begin to create your own solutions. This doesn't preclude the help of a clinician – however only 'you' can choose to put solutions into effect.

➤ Chunk down – Solutions thinkers take the big picture and chunk it down by choosing one area to focus their attention on. They commit to taking the necessary first steps before tackling the next priority on the list. They begin to feel bigger than the problem – it literally diminishes in size – and consequently they feel more in control. Try this. Make a picture of a worry that you had that was overwhelming and literally shrink it into the distance making it smaller and smaller. Notice how much more in control you feel.

➤ Procedures for each option – All solutions require effective procedures – the steps, strategies and the know-how to put it all into effect. Clinicians may help people unearth and use previously hidden resources from other life contexts. They may help them to follow a plan or blueprint that other successful achievers have used in similar situations. They may need to get them to commit to learning new skills. This is where the 'rubber hits the road' and may well be the most important part of a solutions focus.

Let's once more take our smoker who is keen to stop. They focus on the positive benefits of stopping smoking – healthier lungs, improved fitness, more money (towards). They name a date for stopping and commit to it (proactive). When people offer them a cigarette they decline (internal locus). They choose one area at a time to give their commitment to – work, home etc. (chunk down). They may use several different strategies – say, gum, patches, relaxation – at appropriate times (procedures for each option).

You can use this strategy as a mini-checklist with the other presenting problems listed above to ensure your patients' solutions are well structured.

PROBLEMS TO SOLUTIONS

In each of the succeeding chapters we will tackle various ways of persuading people to let go of problems and make health-improving changes. Here is one useful way to frame the process and begin to ask helpful questions.

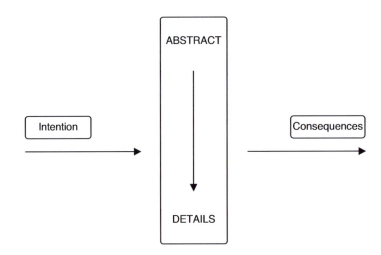

FIGURE 3.1 Problems and solutions

Both problems and solutions can be discussed in abstract or more detailed language. A problem stated as 'I'm depressed' is a high-level abstraction. We need to get more grounded in details about the specifics of the situation, with particular examples of when and where the problem actually occurs. Similarly a solution request of 'I just want to be happy' requires more details of what exactly needs to happen for this to take place. In both instances (problems and solutions) the specifics will include focusing on a particular event and concentrating on the thinking and feeling states that accompany the ongoing, visible behaviour.

All problems have future, potentially negative consequences if not tackled effectively. Solutions have consequences too, sometimes life-changing ones. Also, behind every problem we can unearth a positive intention, what could be called the secondary gain, or better still, the hidden benefits of the situation. For example, the hidden benefit or positive intention of smoking might be to help someone relax if they are feeling harassed and frazzled. We will explore this further in Chapter 8.

For now here are some useful initial questions to consider asking your patients:

Problem strategy

How do you know this is a problem?

What lets you know this is a problem?

How is that affecting you right now?

This recovers more specific information about the problem, what the patient thinks may have caused it and what effect it currently has on their life. If you listen carefully you will elicit how they are structuring the problem and the strategy that keeps it in place (away from, reactive etc.). If you continue to ask this question of each successive answer you will also get quickly to the crux of the issue. Often what is initially presented as a problem is not the 'real' problem. Digging a little deeper may unearth something quite different to what you expect (*see* the next section entitled 'Is the problem really what you think it is?').

For people who are currently oblivious to the effect their current behaviour is having on them (smoking, drinking, overeating, for example) you could ask this variation:

If this were to become a problem, how would you know?

What would let you know that it had become a problem?

These questions crystallise the formation of a problem out of the nebulous background where it currently resides unseen. They give people an opportunity to consider what conditions would have to occur for their current behaviour to become an issue requiring resolution. In these situations it is often important to create a problem to move away from as an initial strategy.

Solution strategy

> *If this problem were solved . . . how would you know?*

> *What would be different . . . About you . . .? The situation . . .?*

> *How will you be as a person once that's happened?*

This information gives you (and them) the particular details about how specifically the future needs to be different from the past, and what might need to take place to get there intact. If you listen carefully you can ensure they are structuring the solution effectively (towards, proactive etc.). It is important to find out what particular, observable behaviours they will be carrying out instead, as well as how they are thinking and feeling differently when they have what they really want.

Discriminatory strategy

> *How do you know what to do to get there?*

> *What skills and strategies will you use?*

Whenever a person wants to make changes they need to know which of their many skills and resources will best fit and match the circumstances. These questions will help you decide whether they do indeed have the necessary skills and how confident they are in using them. Of course there may be a skills gap. You may have to help them unearth various abilities and talents from other life contexts. You may even have to teach them some new skills. Discriminating in this way finds the right tool for the task in hand.

These questions are disarmingly simple yet can get right to the heart of any change issues. I suggest you begin to incorporate them in as many consultations as possible.

IS THE PROBLEM REALLY WHAT YOU THINK IT IS?

On the face of it, when people bring their problems to the consulting room we may be seduced into thinking that this is the issue that needs to be fixed. If only I didn't smoke, drink, eat too much, spend too much money, take drugs, take too little exercise, watch too much television, not take my medication, not love my husband, dislike my job etc., then things would be fine. As clinicians we then help develop strategies to tackle the problem behaviour. We have behavioural programmes to reduce drinking, stop smoking, lose weight and myriads more. However we may be totally missing the mark.

Sometimes, perhaps more often than not, tackling the errant behaviours may *not* solve the real problem at all. Most problems have one thing in common. They are usually our best current method for escaping from negative feelings which we can't handle. Many people have not learned healthy ways to deal with difficult emotions and situations – or difficult people. We may not have been brought up in a way that has naturally taught us negotiation and mediation skills, assertiveness training, socialisation skills, the ability to compartmentalise negative feelings, how to deal effectively with the frustrations of not getting what we want in life and so on.

Our remedies are to reach for our 'drug of choice' to tranquillise the negative feelings away and soothe our hurt egos. If we engage in a new behavioural change programme that takes our comfort blanket away from us we may be left once more in the open, laid bare to the hurts but unable to do anything about it. This is like being caught between the devil and the deep blue sea – better the devil you know.

For some people there is a common belief that underlies and triggers the negative feelings that result in problem behaviour. That is often voiced as one or another variation of 'I'm just not good enough'. This statement of belief, almost always a surviving remnant of early childhood experiences, is a key determinant of the oft times low or poor self-esteem that drives what are essentially self-harming behaviours. What can we do about this? Well, the first thing is simply to keep it in mind in any individual's change process. A key question to ask yourself is:

> What is the real issue here . . . is it the behaviour . . . or something else?

A problem is the end result of a series of thinking, feeling and behavioural strategies. It is not a reified thing in its own right but we often treat it as if it were written immutably on a tablet of stone. Once we start to view problems as the end result of a process with a beginning, middle and end point, we can track the process far enough back to get to a pivotal intervention point. Another key question to keep in mind is:

> What sequence of processes (thinking, feeling, behaving) had to happen for this problem to be the end result?

When you start thinking in this way you prevent yourself joining your patient and sharing the stuck feelings that surround the problem issue. There really is no point in both of you getting mired in the negativity. It is important that you get enough distance to give you a wider perspective of the train of events that have led to the current situation. Staying out of the tunnel vision that focuses on premature problem solving allows you to divert the train at its head rather than trying to derail the rear carriages only.

Box 3.1 Awareness-raising questions

Here are some more questions to help you identify the process behind the problem.

What's really going on here . . .?
What's the bigger picture that this is part of . . .?
What sequences of repeated thoughts, feelings and behaviours keep recurring . . .?
What underlying belief is driving the show . . .?
What is really triggering this issue . . .?
What choice points can I identify that will change the direction . . .?
Where can I intervene most effectively . . .?
Where is the smallest point of intervention with the most leverage . . .?

GOING WHERE THE PROBLEM ISN'T . . .

You rarely find a solution by focusing entirely on the problem. By so doing you are likely to remain enmeshed in the kinds of thinking that brought the issue about, and maintain it. The feelings, emotions and states that surround a problem situation are often very negative (e.g. depression). Staying in them for any length of time is likely to lead to feeling stuck, immobile and with no apparent way out. Major impediments to change include fear, exhaustion, internal and external conflict, feeling scattered and directionless and, in particular, overwhelm. We need to change focus and look elsewhere.

Solution spaces

Solution spaces – times and places where the problem doesn't occur – arise every day in our patients' lives almost without notice. People always have times during their day when they are, at least temporarily, not thinking about their issue because they are thinking or doing something different instead. Their attention is focused elsewhere. Someone who is depressed may still get engrossed in their favourite television show and for half an hour or more may not think of their depression. People can also forget to have their problem when in the shower, at the supermarket, reading a book, dancing, making love or doing any one of myriad other things instead.

Certain places may make the behaviour untenable for a period of time. Smokers who go on transatlantic flights have to do without a cigarette for nine hours or more. In the UK there is now a smoking ban in public places and again people have to temper their behaviours accordingly. It is very useful to seek out these places and times and find out just exactly how someone was able to cope. What did they actually do when temptation struck but they couldn't follow through on their habitual behaviours?

Counterexamples

It is also worthwhile seeking counterexamples – times when the problem should have occurred but didn't. Perhaps someone turned down a drink or a cigarette. Maybe they felt the urge to binge eat but on this occasion they didn't follow through. Perhaps they were doing another behaviour that was incompatible with the problem behaviour. It is hard to smoke or eat when you are engaged in exercise or doing something that fully occupies your hands.

These are all very important instances and they happen whatever presenting problem we focus on. Within them lie the seeds of naturally occurring mental and physical strategies that this particular individual has used to good effect. Paying attention to how this has come about can bring these strategies to awareness and allow them to be used with intention in challenging times.

Think of times when you should have had your problem behaviour but didn't, and times and places when it doesn't occur at all. Get a specific example in mind, a real event, and answer the following questions.

Box 3.2 Going where the problem isn't: solution space questions

Where are you located on these occasions?
How does this specific event come about?
What is actually happening at these times?
What are you focusing on instead?
What are you thinking and feeling then?
What are you doing physically in those moments?
How can you use what you've learned intentionally in the future?

The knowledge gained from these questions can help you devise a plan of action that encompasses people's natural strategies – what works best for them as unique individuals when their problem temporarily ceases to exist. They can help you fine-tune the change process so that tailor-made solutions can dovetail more easily into their normal way of life.

Interventions that give people back an internal locus of control are often the prime determinants of lasting change. Identifying and dealing with the key emotions that serve to obfuscate the issue can often disperse the fog and allow us to see more clearly the required action steps. One of the quickest ways to raise self-esteem is either to show someone that they actually do have the necessary skills hidden away in another context or to help them rapidly acquire, assimilate and master those which are required in their particular situation. There are many examples of 'model' individuals who do have the necessary skill sets and the steps they use have been codified and written down in easy-to-use formats.

Another very useful way of increasing internal locus of control is to get people in touch with their signature strengths so they can bring them to bear in present circumstances. The various exercises in Chapter 9 help people to bring to mind personal past achievements and their associated states of mind and body which bolster self-esteem. When people feel good about themselves, when they love and appreciate themselves for who they really are at the deepest level, when they recognise that they can take effective action on their own behalf to resolve underlying issues, then recourse to problem behaviour becomes moot – it is no longer required.

Chapter 3 outline summary

Structure and content
- *Content* – storyline or current narrative that the patient uses to explain and make some sense out of what is happening to them
- *Structure* – the repetitive thinking, feeling and behavioural patterns through which the content flows

Problem structure
- *Away from* – what's wrong/not wanted
- *Reactive* – paralysis by analysis/rumination
- *External locus of control* – learned helplessness
- *Chunked up* – overwhelming BIG picture
- *Options with no procedures* – don't know HOW to proceed

Solution structure
- *Towards* – what you really want to have happen instead
- *Proactive* – take action
- *Internal locus of control* – take responsibility for making changes
- *Chunked down* – choose one area to focus attention on
- *Procedure for each option* – steps, strategies and know-how

Problems to solutions

- *Problem strategy*
  - How do you know this is a problem?
  - What lets you know this is a problem?
  - If this were to become a problem, how would you know?
- *Solution strategy*
  - If this problem were solved, how would you know?
  - What would be different . . . About you? . . .The situation?
- *Discriminatory strategy*
  - How do you know what to do to get there?
  - What resources/skills/strategies will you use?

Is the problem really what you think it is?

Problem behaviours are often our best current method for escaping from underlying negative emotions and are substitutes for our lack of skills in various areas (assertiveness, relationships, problem solving, negotiation, mediation, compartmentalisation etc.)

- What is the real issue here . . . the problem behaviour . . . or something else underlying it?
- What sequence of processes (thinking, feeling, behaving) had to happen for this problem to be the end result?
- Ask the other awareness raising questions

Going where the problem isn't . . .

- *Solution spaces*
  - times and places where the problem doesn't occur
- *Counterexamples*
  - times and places when the problem should have occurred but didn't

Ask solution space questions to identify the naturally occurring mental and physical strategies that people use in these contexts so they can be utilised intentionally in the problem area.

CHAPTER 4

Assessing importance, confidence and readiness for change

HOW IMPORTANT IS IT FOR YOU TO CHANGE?

This is an important question. Some patients say they really want to change but when push comes to shove, it's not the most significant thing in their life currently and falls well down their list of priorities. Others have change as a high priority but lack the confidence to do so. Importance is connected to our values, the meanings in life that we find deeply significant and our current priorities. Confidence, on the other hand, reflects our degree of certainty that the skills we have are adequate to the task we currently face. Both are required to work together for change to occur. You can get an idea of where people are at by asking a scaling question from 1 to 10, where level 1 is low importance or confidence and level 10 is high.

(On a scale of 1–10)

How important is it for you to make this change . . .?

How confident are you that you could make this change if you really want to . . .?

Here is a simple grid of the various response combinations (*see* Figure 4.1) that shows quite clearly where the work needs to be done. Groups 1 and 2 do not currently rate the importance of changing very highly so it is unlikely to happen. In Group 3, perceived importance is high though confidence is low. What they need is an effective strategy for change which they believe can work for them, thus increasing their perceived self-efficacy. This is a similar situation in Group 1 also, though for them it may be of more value to work on increasing importance first.

In this simplistic model Group 4 seems to be the most favourably disposed to change occurring. However the real world is often a bit different to the model we make of it. For Group 4, changing will depend on how *ready* they are to engage in the process. Despite importance and confidence being high, their energies may be so fully occupied with current life demands that change has a lower priority in the overall scheme of things at this time. The question here then is all about timing: *when?*

As a clinician, please keep in mind the following question in every consultation:

> *How ready is this particular person to make changes?*

Importance and confidence interact in more complex and interdependent ways. For some people it may be that until they first develop the confidence that they have the necessary skills then they cannot contemplate importance at all (Group 1). They may feel quite hopeless. For others (Group 3), they may be in a very distressing situation where they rate importance extremely highly but see the goal as way beyond their reach because they don't have the skills. They feel helpless, like a rabbit caught in the headlights of an oncoming personal disaster.

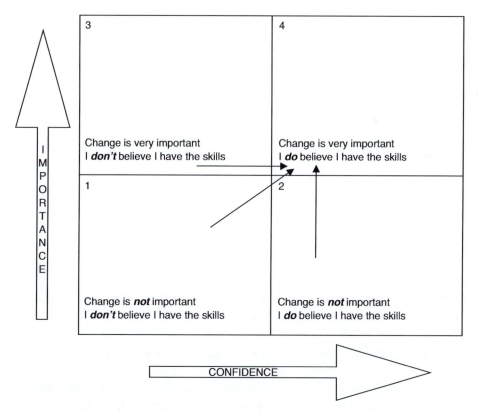

FIGURE 4.1 Assessing importance and confidence

Raising the scaling numbers

Whichever number your patient's current rating is at for importance, confidence is always a good place to start. The tendency is for clinicians to ask: 'Why are you at a 3 and not at a 5?' This is not terribly useful and may, through psychological reactance, keep the situation stuck. Essentially it tells someone that they are inadequate to the task and have failed to reach some external standard. It tends to invoke a negative comparison of self-to-other rather than a positive one of self-to-self. More useful is to say the following:

>*You're at a 3 . . . that's great . . . tell me why it's a 3 and not a 1 . . .*

Starting with this kind of positive comparison from self now to self in the past aids in the further development of rapport and the therapeutic alliance. It is the opposite of what most people expect and is delightfully wrong-footing in a constructive and helpful way. It simultaneously asks the patient to search for and name the fledgling resources and skills of which they may have been completely unaware. Once named, an opportunity arises to further elucidate and strengthen them, and then put them to work. It encourages patients to begin a very useful strategy of making positive comparisons and supports increasing self-efficacy. You can then follow up with:

>*So, what would a 4 look like . . .?*

Then:

>*And what would need to happen for you to be able to move there . . .?*

By further defining the details of what moving to a 4 encompasses – the specific, observable behaviours and actions – you are covertly setting it as an achievable goal. You are also helping them delineate the few simple steps they can take along the pathway they are constructing for themselves. If they own the process they are more likely to take the steps.

This is incremental change at its very best: a very small nudge resulting in one or two bite-size steps that provides both the direction and the momentum for further gains. You can use this strategy over and over again. And by utilising psychological reactance once more you can finish by saying:

>*. . . But don't take any steps until you're absolutely ready . . .*

This prevents them from experiencing you as pushing them to take action to which they might respond negatively. It puts the ball directly back in their court and gives them complete control of whether or not they engage in the first steps.

It can be very tempting to give someone a helpful shove if you perceive them as teetering on the brink. In a word – don't. You are far more likely to entice them forwards by appearing to hold them back – just a little.

Remember this principle: Less equals more.

Response–ability

It is worthwhile saying a little bit more about 'response-ability' and responsibility. When people are 'response-able' they can choose their response to whatever is happening in their life. We cannot control all of life's circumstances. In fact we often naively believe we have much more control and certainty over future events than we really do – until disaster strikes. At that point we can either adopt the identity of victim status, which may attract lots of attention ('Oh you poor thing to have that happen to you, it must be so awful') but potentially leaves us even more mired in the problem. Or, we can recognise that no matter what is happening right now we always have choices about how we respond and what we can do.

Some people say we are always responsible for every single one of our actions – that is, called to account as the primary cause, motive or agent. Yet when it comes to thinking about problems, many people equate this with a blame frame – you are at fault in some way. This kind of thinking goes along the lines of: if we are truly responsible for this problem then we must have caused or created it in some way and therefore we are to blame . . . guilty of the offence. This is an added burden of negative emotion that potentially makes the situation even harder to bear.

In essence we are doing the best we can, minute-to-minute, day-by-day, with the resources we have available to us. If we could have made changes in the past and done things differently then we would have. What is done is done, and continuing to beat ourselves up over what has already happened is fruitless. What we *are* responsible for is making the choice to do something about our habitual, knee-jerk, conditioned reflex reactions so that we can respond differently here and now and on into the future – that is, be response-able.

When people start to take this kind of response-ability for themselves they begin to markedly increase their inner locus of control whilst recognising, paradoxically, that there are fewer things in the outside world they can truly control. Things such as other individuals' thoughts, beliefs, values, actions and behaviours (spouse, children, work colleagues etc.), the state of the economy, political decisions and even the weather. This can be a very liberating experience – letting go of controlling the uncontrollable.

On the other hand it also puts the responsibility for making change happen back exactly where it belongs, one hundred per cent, fully and completely into patients' hands. This does not absolve us as clinicians from utilising our skills to the maximum in persuading our patients to make changes. However, we are *not* responsible for their making the change – they are. If, however, you do assume this kind of responsibility for your patient then you are in great danger of creating a co-dependent relationship. Rescuing people may have many psychological pay-offs and give many warm fuzzy inner feelings but the main casualty is independence – both yours and theirs. Throughout *Persuasion in* Clinical *Practice* you will find many ways to use your skills with integrity and promote co-independence instead.

Chapter 4 outline summary

Importance, confidence and readiness

- *Importance* – a value judgment about worth, degree of priority
- *Confidence* – belief in one's capabilities to act
- *Readiness* – a state of mental and physical preparedness to take action

Scaling questions

(On a scale of 1–10)

How important is it for you to make this change?

How confident are you that you could make this change?

How ready are you to take action?

Raising the numbers

(Where X is the current number they're at)

You're at X . . . that's great . . . tell me why it's X and not X-1 or X-2?

What would X+1 look like?

And what would need to happen for you to move there?

Responsibility and response-ability

- *Responsibility* – called to account as the primary cause, motive or agent . . . often used in a blaming fashion implying control of the uncontrollable
- *Response-ability* – making the choice to respond differently here and now to old conditioned reflexes and behaviours

Present and curious

The clinician from hell is not a pretty sight to behold – worse still to consult with. You may have been in the presence of one or more during your clinical lifetime. There are many different types, ranging from the more austere authoritarian, a cold fish with poor rapport skills, to the overempathisers who personally feel every single bit of pain their patient goes through – and want to rescue them to boot. Whilst both are at different ends of the spectrum their overall effect is similar – disenfranchised patients.

Although something of a caricature, the archetypical austere clinician remains very distant from patients and may seem to make clinical pronouncements from an ivory tower. In some ways this is quite paternalistic, taking full responsibility for prescribing the correct course of action for the particular condition with scant regard for patient input. In fact the patient may be blamed, overtly or covertly, for causing their problem in the first place. It is as if there is only one right way to get the required result and the patient's duty is to get on with taking the prescription – they know all the answers. Next please!

Whilst empathic communication is important, it can certainly be overdone. Overempathisers feel every stumble, trip and blow of the patient's narrative journey. They deeply feel for the other person's pain and want to rescue them from it. Whilst this is an important driver for many who enter the clinical field it can become a liability if taken too far – especially if they assume responsibility for both the patient's problem and getting the result for them. Whereas the austere authoritarian has rigid personal boundaries, the overempathiser may appear to have no boundaries at all. This is a recipe for co-dependency and clinician burnout.

Of course clinicians like this don't exist, do they? However, I'm certain we can all recognise times when we may have inadvertently and temporarily adopted some aspects of those clinical styles with less than optimal results. It is easy to fall into them, especially when we feel harassed, overwhelmed, struggling for time and just simply overloaded. So just what are the kinds of qualities we are looking for instead in a clinician?

Good clinicians respect you as a unique individual in your own right. They recognise that you're having a hard time but that you, as a whole person, are so much more than your current difficulties. They have the ability to separate out what you do (your behaviours) from who you are (your identity). They don't have a 'one-size fits all' approach. They tend to engage you in finding the kinds of answers that best fit your situation. Of course to do that they need to ask great questions . . . and give enough space for your responses.

They are able to set frames, differentiating their patient's narrative from the underlying processes and repetitive patterns. They look for what is already working well in someone's life rather than being tunnel-visioned and solely addressing the problem. Good clinicians pay attention to the nuances of the unfolding experience – both verbally and non-verbally. They are curious about what is currently happening, completely present to the occurrence. Eschewing the one right answer, they help you explore both what you want and how you will get there. They hold you accountable for agreements and commitments you make with yourself and they engage you in the states of mind and body that facilitate the change process.

Key to this kind of working with patients are two ways of being: *present and curious.* We will explore each in turn and develop your ability to access these states with more frequency and depth.

BEING PRESENT

When you are completely present in the here and now you are open and available to what is happening in this current moment – both for you and your patients. When you focus your attention in this way, thoughts of the past and future recede into the distance. It is as if you have entered a timeless spaciousness. You may even have a sense of everything slowing down, your eyesight becoming keener and your hearing sharpened.

You become more attuned to the nuances of the interaction with your patient. You are able to notice subtle non-verbal clues; changes in voice pitch and tempo, direction of eye gaze, repetitive mini-gestures, breathing patterns, throat clearings and pauses and the incongruities at play within the mixed messages being presented. This information has always been there – the trouble is, you have often been anywhere else but present to it.

So, where do you go to when you're not altogether here, not really present? There are several ways you can escape from the here and now. You may be off in a past memory, of good times or misery. This may have been triggered by something this person said or may simply be your favourite way of disengaging. Perhaps they remind you of someone you dislike or you remember past fruitless consultations with them. When people are depressed or overwhelmed they are often stuck in repetitive negative ruminations of past hurts.

You can also escape into the future. You may be pleasantly anticipating coffee or lunch or perhaps worrying that you will be terribly late for both. When people are anxious – and clinicians are not immune – they are often worrying about possible off-putting future consequences that loom so large as to obscure all else. We can also spend much time looking forward to the end of this particular consultation if we are already running late. Playing catch-up is not a pleasant feeling.

It is possible to be cut off in a here and now that is not shared with the patient. Perhaps you are attending to inputting data into a computer that is always crying out greedily to be fed. Maybe you are simply distracted or preoccupied with something else happening concurrently – the screaming child in the waiting room. Perhaps you are muttering under your breath some curses and oaths in true Victor Meldrew fashion and hoping, like some of my colleagues have confided, that you haven't said anything out loud.

Many clinicians initially resist being completely present because they think they may lose control of the consultation. Or worse still, that consulting in this way will prolong the consultation and make them run even more behind time. Usually the reverse is true. When you are paying complete attention to what is happening right now, your enhanced patient-clinician connection and increased sensory acuity helps you get more rapidly to the roots of the current issue. You actually get to make best use of the time available. And what's more, your patients really appreciate the depth of rapport attained – the therapeutic alliance being an important change tool in its own right (*see* page 11).

Here are some questions that will help you get back in touch with the qualities associated with being present. Exploring your experience in this way will help you to reaccess this state more easily. Think of three different times and contexts when you have been fully present to your ongoing experience, and explore each in turn.

Box 5.1 What's it like when you are present?

Where were you when you were experiencing this?
Were you alone or in company?
What were you doing – what were you focusing on?
What's it like when you are fully present – what does it feel like in your body?
What happens to your vision when you're like this?
What happens to your hearing?
What qualities enable you to be this way?
What interferes with being this way?
How can you be more fully present when you are consulting – what trigger will you use to remind you of this state?

When you explore experiences in this way you are examining just how you create the states of mind and body that go along with the word label 'present'. Mostly this has been out of your conscious awareness. Yet thinking about it again will take you back into the very same thoughts, feelings and behaviours as the original event. You will find that when you pay attention in the same way again you will begin to automatically trigger this way of being once more – this time when it will be even more useful – in the consultation itself.

Here are some other things you can explore which will help you attune more effectively to the present moment.

Box 5.2 Ways of attuning to the present

- Look at any objects around you and trace their edges and borders in your mind's eye.
- Pay attention to the shape of the space between two or more objects.
- Notice how they relate to one another (height, depth, foreground, background).
- Notice where the light reflects and the size and shape of the shadows.
- If you are with someone (or watching television), notice the changing shapes of the shadows on their face as they speak.
- Listen to the tempo of their speech, the loudness and softness, and any pauses.
- Listen to all the sounds around you and notice how many you can hear.
- Pay attention to the background silence out of which each sound arises and falls.
- As you look straight ahead, simultaneously notice what you can see out of the corners of each eye – without moving your head.
- Pretend that you can 'soften' your eyes and see 360 degrees all around.

BEING CURIOUS

Have you ever wondered what it would be like if you became more curious about your patients? What would happen if you began to get interested in not only what wasn't working in their life, but also what was? Curiosity is an expectant state – you don't know the answers . . . yet you want to find out. It is an open and inviting state – accepting of what is, with an undercurrent of inquisitiveness and enquiry. Rather than taking things at face value you gently probe and examine what lies below the surface. There are no definite rights and wrongs, just a genuine interest in how the puzzle presented to you fits together.

When you are curious about someone's experience in this way, you suspend your absolute judgment for a time and see what evolves. You ask questions about how this particular individual views their own situation and what intuitions they may have about what can resolve it. Rather than dismissing these out of hand, you hold them up for examination so that perhaps a different perspective can arise. This is an inductive process – you don't know beforehand what will come up. It is sometimes surprising, even life-changing. When people feel attended to with genuine curiosity, they open up to the possibility that maybe, just maybe, things can turn out differently.

Rather than displaying curiosity we may fall into the trap of making snap clinical judgments. If we have been trained in hard science and deductive reasoning it is challenging to suspend our traditional thinking patterns and allow space for something else – especially when time may be at a premium. There is a certain comfort in being 'right', and a major discomfort in being 'wrong'. When we judge the correctness of experience in this way we compartmentalise it, put it in a box and throw away the key. We prescribe the rote solutions that we feel we ought to, and feel uneasy about opening a veritable Pandora's box.

How do you tolerate ambiguity, uncertainty and even confusion? The degree to which you can do this is a measure of your ability to remain curious. Most of us dislike the uncomfortable feelings that confusion brings and want to bring them swiftly to an end. I suspect that this is partially due to an age regression phenomenon. When we are confused, not knowing what to do can make us feel like a helpless child again. We want to push this seemingly negative state away. We crave the stability that feeling certain gives us – a feeling of being in control.

When, instead, we approach ambiguity, uncertainty and confusion from a place of curiosity, suspending the need for an instant answer or a quick fix, then we can begin to tease out the various strands of intertwined information. If we can tolerate the not-knowing for a period of time and liken it to doing a crossword puzzle or jigsaw instead, then we may well be rewarded with a completely different, and eminently useful, new perspective. Curiosity holds the key.

Here are some questions that will help you get back in touch with the qualities associated with being curious. Exploring your experience in this way will help you to reaccess this state more easily. Think of three different times and contexts when you have been full of curiosity, wonderment, even an expectant sense of awe about your ongoing experience. Explore each in turn using the questions below.

Box 5.3 What's it like when you are curious?

Where were you when you were experiencing this?

Were you alone or in company?

What were you doing – what were you focusing on?

What's it like when you are really curious – what does it feel like in your body?

What happens to your vision when you're like this?
What happens to your hearing?
What qualities enable you to be this way?
What interferes with being this way?
How can you be more curious when you are consulting – what trigger will you use to remind you of this state?

You will find that, in exactly the same way as you explored being present, the feeling states associated with curiosity will take you back into similar thoughts and behaviours as if you were in the original events themselves. Once again, by paying attention to your ongoing experience, you will uncover the seemingly automatic responses that trigger this state in the here and now. You can now plan to use this in your next series of consultations – when appropriate.

Here are some other things you can explore to further develop your curiosity.

Box 5.4 Developing curiosity

Pick up an everyday object such as a stone or a leaf. Simply look at it for five minutes from different angles noticing the patterns, colours, light and shadows.

Listen to some familiar music. What feeling is the composer trying to elicit?

Next time you are having a leisurely coffee or lunch, pay attention to someone you don't know very well. Ask yourself the following questions . . .

I wonder what things they like . . .?
I wonder what motivates them each day . . .?
I wonder what they are really passionate about . . .?
Are they right- or left-handed . . .?
What might they be thinking right now . . .?
What does the way they dress tell me about their values . . .?
Are they sporty or sedentary . . .?

CONGRUENCE AND INCONGRUENCE

The ability to know whether someone is acting congruently or incongruently is pivotal to persuasion and change processes. Incongruence is a signal of an out-of-awareness conflict. This is when there is a difference between how you are presenting yourself to the world and what is actually happening inside you. It is the basis for many symptoms and unresolved problems. It is particularly common in the stage of resolving ambivalence when someone may be in two minds about whether to change . . . or not. Incongruence can be thought of as the 'but' in 'yes, but . . .' and may be spoken or remain unspoken, appearing non-verbally as asymmetrical postures and gestures.

Congruence, on the other hand, is when you are 'all of a piece'. This is when how you are feeling on the inside matches what you are presenting on the outside. Your words, voice tone, posture and gestures are all in sync. When people are truly aligned and committed to some venture, you can see this quite clearly in their body language which tends to be symmetrical.

Notice how you feel when you engage in the two experiences below.

Box 5.5 Your incongruence signal

Check out your feelings when:

- You remember getting a present from someone and you didn't want it or like it . . . yet you had to open it in front of them and pretend that you did.
- You remember telling someone that you would do something you didn't want to do and resented being asked to do . . . such as working late or seeing an extra patient.

Box 5.6 Your congruence signal

Check out your feelings when:

- You remember being determined to do something, you did it, and looking back it is still a good decision today.
- You remember doing something really well, you know you did it well and someone said 'well done!'

Identifying these signals for yourself can be very helpful in distinguishing incongruence in both you and your patients. When you are in rapport with someone and you begin to feel confused, puzzled or ill at ease, then you can use this signal to alert you to step back and seek more information before making a decision about what to do next. The clearer you are about your own signals for congruence and incongruence the more easily you will be able to pick up on patients' spoken and unspoken incongruities.

There is often a lot of incongruence present in the 'resolving ambivalence' phase. This is because the person is in two minds about what to do. The incongruence may be expressed simultaneously when the verbal and non-verbal communication is clearly at odds right here and now. It might be expressed sequentially when at one time they feel committed to taking the next step yet at another time they fail to actually do what they promised.

This is usually a sign that some information is missing. For example, they may want to make a change but not know *what* to do or *how* to do it. It may signal a conflict between beliefs and values – they may have the skills but the change is not a high enough priority right now. Sometimes there is hesitation because to really make the change may not fit with their sense of self – it would be like becoming another person altogether. Sensitively exploring this information gap can help resolution occur more ecologically.

Here are some typical expressions of incongruence to listen out for.

Box 5.7 Typical incongruence in action

Yes I'll try that . . . but . . .

On the one hand what you're saying makes sense . . .

Yes I think I can do that . . . (said with a sigh)

I'll give it my best shot . . . (simultaneous shake of the head)

I can see what I need to do . . . it just doesn't feel right . . .

When conflicts have been resolved, people become more congruent, aligned and committed to the result they want to obtain. This is clear in their body language and you can sense this as a clinician because you will experience your own feelings of congruence simultaneously. In fact, if you do not get this feeling you should be very wary about nudging them into the next stage. Developing your expertise in reading these signals is therefore vital to monitoring the change process. Because ambivalence can occur in any of the stages of change, honing your sensory acuity in this way will allow your patients a smoother navigation to where they want to go.

Chapter 5 outline summary

Being present

- Open and available to what is happening right now
- Thoughts of past and future recede
- A feeling of timeless spaciousness
- Increased sensory acuity . . . noticing nuances of non-verbal communication
- Deepening of rapport

A quick way to enter this state is to pretend that you can 'soften' your eyes and see 360 degrees all around

Being curious

- An open and inviting state
- A sense of underlying inquisitiveness and enquiry
- Suspension of judgment
- Increased toleration of ambiguity, uncertainty and confusion
- An inductive process of examining different perspectives

A quick way to enter this state is to ask yourself questions beginning with 'I wonder . . .'

Being congruent

- A feeling of being 'all of a piece'
- Words, voice tone, posture and gesture all in sync
- Alignment of values, goal and behaviours
- Fully committed to the task in hand

Be alert for signals of congruence when discussing management plans and next steps

Being incongruent

- A signal of an out-of-awareness conflict
- Ambivalent and being in 'two minds'
- Asymmetry of posture, gesture, voice tone and words
- The 'but' in 'Yes, but . . .'

Incongruence is often a signal of lack of information, especially about 'what' to do and 'how' to do it

Avoiding roadblocks

As clinicians we have to be very wary of the assumptions we often unwittingly make about a particular person's motivation for change. We do the job we do because we place a high premium on health and may presume, mistakenly, that others do too. We know the types of behavioural change that would be of most benefit so it is very easy to imply overtly or covertly that this person *ought* to make changes right now. We might even believe that they really *want* to change without doing one important thing – checking with them first. Frustrating as it may initially seem, some people are happy to glory on in the same vein day after day.

Deciding to make a change is a process, not an all-or-nothing, one-time event. Similarly, motivation to change can be non-existent on some days, very high on others and fluctuate in between during the rest of the time. Sometimes we may feel like we've failed if this person doesn't make the commitment to change today. We may even write them off as 'no-hopers' and convey that attitude in subsequent consultations – a self-fulfilling prophecy. It is important to keep in mind, however, that although now may not be the right time, there are many other opportunities when the ebb and flow of motivation and the rise and fall of readiness for change may coincide propitiously. In persuasion for change, timing is all.

Some clinicians believe that taking a hard-line, tough love approach is always best. As the expert they are there to impart their views and advice (nay, commands) on what you ought to do next. If you have ever been on the receiving end of this type of consultation you will know that it is unlikely to be effective. Very occasionally it can hit the nail on the head and be just what the doctor ordered. Mostly, though, it is a prime tool for generating massive resistance and major roadblocks. Whilst every behavioural approach is useful in some circumstances, and flexibility is often the name of the game, it is wise to keep the heavy hand mostly in your back pocket.

Your expertise is not irrelevant. It is just that, in the general scheme of things, telling people what to do is very unlikely to help them develop and internalise the skills they need to make change permanent. Persuasion is not coercion. It is more of a negotiation where, although the patient is ultimately in charge of where they want to go, you are there to give them helpful nudges in the right direction, and be responsible for overseeing the process of change. Remember too, though, that negotiation is only one end of the spectrum of tools for intervention – not the be-all and end-all.

In the next section we will discuss four of the major roadblocks to avoid before moving on to some verbal and non-verbal tools you can use instead.

FOUR MAJOR ROADBLOCKS

Why do roadblocks exist? Mostly they are conditioned reflexes built up over many years of clinical practice. A large number of clinicians are motivated by helping people get out of difficult situations – for many it is their *raison d'être*. When you know what the potential solutions may be, you want to rescue as many as possible from their plight. Unfortunately this 'rescuing' has a downside.

By assuming the responsibility of solving people's issues for them you can increase the feeling that they are helpless victims not only of problems but also solutions. You can reinforce a state of learned helplessness – instilling the belief that they don't have the skills to help themselves. If a similar issue crops up again, rather than being able to deal with it effectively, they have to return to a more powerful 'authority' to get fixed. This can breed resentment and frustration.

Of course resentment and frustration are no strangers to the clinician either. When people return over and over again as a hapless victim with the same unresolved issues it's easy to fall into blame mode and play the persecutor card. Suppressed anger may boil over with accusations of fault, culpability and lack of responsibility for actions. The ensuing pangs of guilt may then start the rescue cycle over again.

The four roadblocks described below have all the above features in common.

Prescribing solutions

If you prematurely prescribe solutions without taking the time to give your patient an opportunity to fully say their piece, feel that you have understood their predicament or engage their problem-solving capacities, then you are doing them a disservice. And not only that, they may also sense that you are not really fully considering their situation and may even feel put down, lectured to or even hectored. As a consequence they might think they are being pushed into a hasty or impulsive decision. At worst, you may leave them feeling quite stupid and even more out of touch with whatever problem-solving abilities they possess.

Here are the kinds of things you may catch yourself saying impulsively:

Why don't you just do this instead . . . I'm sure it will help . . .

I've seen this before . . . this is what you need to do . . .

If you continue like this you'll only make things worse . . . research shows . . .

You need to stop that behaviour now . . . and do this instead . . .

Whilst you may indeed know what kinds of solutions will help their situation it is important that you do enough groundwork to get them to buy into them at a later stage. People rarely act on a prescribed solution unless they feel a major degree of ownership that it's their choice of what to do.

Being judgmental

It is sometimes hard to withhold judgment when someone comes with a repetitive problem that they've not yet resolved. We may be tempted to find fault with them for not having the moral fibre to follow through – or mutter under our breath 'not again'. We may be lured into resorting to blaming or even name-calling. A more intellectual form of blaming goes under the guise of analysing. You tell someone about your theory of their deeper inadequacies which have surfaced as their recurrent issue. This names, blames and shames them by pointing a finger without providing a way out.

When you are in judgmental mode you might find yourself saying:

Well, can't you see how you've caused this yet again . . .?

You really are the architect of your own misfortune . . .

You've been a bit of an idiot again, haven't you . . .?

You do this over and over again because deep down inside you're just needing attention . . .

Sometimes you can say these kinds of things very playfully, with a smile on your face and a wink in your eye, and they may indeed be helpful. Difficulties arise mostly when we say them in a state of congruent vehemence. They are expressions of our own frustrations in the consultation. Getting them out into the open may gave us some short-lived relief. However, it doesn't help the other person very much. What *does* open up a solution space, though, is respectful listening and genuine understanding.

Ignoring

When you are busy it's very easy to ignore what someone is telling you: not the superficial words as such, but the underlying emotional tones and internal conflicts. Surface listening is akin to preaching platitudes. In a nutshell, you skim over what's presented and offer clichéd responses – a bit like being at a cocktail party. It seems like you're paying attention, but you're not really. You leave the other person feeling both misunderstood and maybe even chastised. They may not say any more about the issue yet inside they may still be fermenting.

When you are ignoring someone you are likely to be using the following phrases:

Don't worry, I'm sure you'll find a way round it as usual . . .

I know it's a bit tough just now but a good person like you will find a way to deal with it . . .

Never mind, things have a habit of working out for the best in the end . . .

I'm sure there are other things in life you can focus on instead . . .

Platitudes may stop people talking about their problem but that doesn't stop them worrying. At best it lets them know not to knock on your door again – at least not with this issue. At worst any inner conflict remains unresolved. Once again, respectful listening bites the dust.

Cross-examining

Being met with a barrage of questions can seem like an inquisitorial interrogation – the Spanish Inquisition. This is especially so if the questions are fired off with little space for an adequate answer. Rather than helping people open up about what is troubling them and what they'd like to do instead, it usually leads to closing down behaviour, battening down the defensive hatches, and even distraction and confusion. Cross-examining (and I use the word 'cross' advisedly) helps you keep charge of the conversation at the expense of curtailing the bringing to bear of the other person's problem-solving skills.

You might just find yourself using the following words:

Why on earth did you do that . . .?

Why haven't you sorted this out previously . . .?

Don't you have the ability to do something about this yourself . . .?

Did you tell him/her exactly what you wanted . . .?

To do cross-examining well, you need to fire off your next question before they've finished answering the last one. Any answers that are generated tend to be of the defensive variety rather than solution-focused.

In the main, helping clinicians don't deliberately use these roadblocks. Often they are actually trying to give of their best in challenging circumstances. No one likes the feeling of being out of control. These responses are often a knee-jerk strategy to actually help control the information flow, especially when time is of the essence. It sometimes seems that giving up even more time for respectful listening will lead to more pressure. Yet dealing with the right issue at the right time can prevent numerous misunderstandings and be more time-effective in the long run. It's the old adage of making sure the ladder you're climbing is leaning against the right wall.

RESPECTFUL LISTENING

It goes almost without saying then that respectful listening steers clear of the four main roadblocks. But what is it exactly? Respectful listening is the ability to ask open questions, maintain a space for the answers to arise and to attend carefully to what is being said (and not said), both verbally and non-verbally. The receiver not only feels respected, they have a deeper sense of being fully accepted with a mutual understanding of their difficulties. This kind of listening demands a commitment which is amply rewarded by the results. If you want to persuade anyone to make changes you have to start by creating this space.

NON-VERBAL SKILLS

There are a number of body language skills that let people know that you are fully attending to them. Here are the main ones to take on board and use throughout your change consultations.

➤ Sit at a 45-degree angle to the other person. This lets them pay attention to your face and eyes when they need to and also gives an open space between the two of you where they can look away from time to time and 'project' their thoughts.

➤ Maintain a similar eye level if possible and don't gaze at your computer, picture on the wall or out of the window.

➤ Mirroring the speaker's body posture, breathing rate, voice tonality and rate of speech will help deepen your rapport. If they speak fast, speed up a bit yourself and vice versa. Don't mimic too closely – do it respectfully.

➤ Use open postures and gestures and sit with your arms and legs uncrossed.

➤ Nod your head from time to time as they speak but don't overdo it.

➤ Notice their direction of gaze and where it seems to alight when they talk about problems versus solutions. You will notice the state changes associated with each position (e.g. posture, gestures, breathing, head tilts and facial colouring/pallor).

Most of the above behaviours are pretty obvious as they are markers of good attending in almost any conversation. It is often useful to write them out on a series of cards and turn one over just before the next consultation. For the first minute or so you can pay more attention to that skill before letting it drop back out of awareness.

VERBAL SKILLS

The three verbal skills that are most fundamental to effective listening are minimal encouragers, open questions and reflective listening. We will cover the first two here and the third in a section by itself.

Minimal encouragers

These are the grunts and groans, the ums and ahs, the yups, yeahs, sures and rights that let people know that not only are you still awake, you are attending to their ongoing narrative. They are the equivalent of 'go on, I'm still listening'. They neither imply agreement nor disagreement; they simply convey interest. More importantly, in the early stages of storytelling they let the other person hold the floor and continue talking. This is absolutely vital. Studies have shown that many health professionals (especially doctors) interrupt and take over the conversation an average of 17 seconds after the patient has started. Once interrupted, patients never get complete control back again.

Open questions

Open questions are ones that cannot be answered by a simple yes or no. They require elaboration. They ask the receiver to dig a bit deeper under the surface and expose not only the narrative of the current situation but also the emotional overtones and nuances of thought and feelings. These kinds of questions help people to voice and explore their experience, including any ambivalence and inner conflict. By listening to themselves in this way, together with assimilating the clinician's reflective statements, the receiver gets the chance to see in sharp relief, perhaps for the very first time, the detrimental effects of a particular problem behaviour together with possible solutions.

Open questions usually begin with the words 'what' and 'how' and the phrase 'Tell me . . .'. Here are some typical open questions to get people talking about change.

> **Box 6.1 Open questions for change**
> - What concerns you about your current situation . . .?
> - What difficulties have you had in relation to this issue . . .?
> - Tell me how would you like things to be different . . .?
> - What would be the benefits of making this change . . .?
> - How confident are you that you can make this change . . .?
> - What personal strengths can you bring to bear here . . .?
> - How important is making this change to you . . .?
> - What do you think you could do next . . .?

It is often a very useful general strategy to initially keep someone talking by using non-verbal encouragers, and then ask an open question to direct attention towards the topic of change. This will give you plenty of material to use in reflective listening statements and further follow up by utilising the persuasion and change skills described in the other chapters.

REFLECTIVE LISTENING

This is a key skill for opening up a solution space. Our aim is to accurately verbally reflect back to the receiver both the information content of their answers to open questions together with the underlying feelings and emotions that their words and behaviours portray. You are restating the basic meaning of what the other person has said. This is a very useful skill not only in change work but also in negotiations and conflict situations (internal and external). Like all such skills, it can be overused to the point of being annoying, patronising and condescending. Judicious use, though, yields high dividends.

The essence of any reflective response is a 'best guess' as to the meaning of the speaker's words. These words are their attempts to communicate what is really going on for them deep inside. However, the words that someone says may not accurately reflect the underlying meaning they want to get across. And, of course, sometimes people may actually say very little at all. Reflective listening is an attempt to read between the lines of what is said and not said, to accurately intuit, interpret and make sense of each statement. This is mind-reading with one difference – you are continually checking out the veracity of your intuitions with the other person.

There are three main steps to reflective listening:

1   Listen to what the other person has said and ask yourself what the underlying meaning of the communication message was.
2   Put your understanding into a brief statement and say it back to them. Use the same or similar words so that the other person can easily understand

them. When you do this, use a downward inflection at the end of the sentence so it sounds more like a statement than a question.

3   Check with them to see if you have clearly captured the gist of what they originally said.

Initially, when you are learning how to do this, it can seem like hard work and sometimes unnatural. However, it doesn't take much practice for you to be able to integrate this into your normal consulting style and use it when appropriate. From the clinician's point of view, reflective listening doesn't require nearly as much effort as trying desperately to find solutions on the patient's behalf. What it does is allow you to be more fully present in the here and now with an attitude of curiosity which is vital for creating a solution space from which the best fitting answers can arise.

Reflecting skills

There are many different ways in which you can use reflective listening. Each of the ways listed below gets deeper beneath the layers of the surface message and more complex at the same time. What can start off heading in one direction can lead to a completely different place with a more fundamental issue being discussed and resolved.

1   Content: Mainly this is paraphrasing the information that is exchanged in your conversation. This usually remains at a quite superficial level, though it is useful for clarifying that you are in the same ballpark as your patient.

2   Feelings: This is a much deeper response which focuses on how this person is feeling inside *about* the issues under discussion. Examples might be:
   - *You feel ashamed that your drinking has got to this level.*
   - *It was like a punch in the solar plexus when you saw your liver function tests.*
   - *You feel disgusted with yourself that you can't stop smoking.*
   - *On the one hand you really want to stop, but on the other you don't feel you've got the determination to succeed (a double-sided reflection).*

3   Checking intuitions: Sometimes people don't say very much but it is clear from their behaviour, their body language and how they say what they say that they are in the grips of one emotion or another. It is useful to check out your guesses about how they feel in the following way:
   - *You've gone a bit quiet and you seem to be quite sad . . . is that what's happening for you right now . . .?*
   - *You're looking a bit shell-shocked . . . and I wonder if you're feeling a bit confused by all this . . .?*
   - *You're not saying very much . . . but from how you look I wonder if you're feeling angry inside . . . could that be the case?*

4   Summarising and signposting: Summarising is when you take a number of statements over a period of time and restate them to ensure you have agreement before going on to the next step. Signposting is when you say what the possible next steps could be and invite them to choose what they'd like to do. Some examples:

- *So you've been thinking about stopping smoking for several months now . . . you've had two unsuccessful attempts in the past . . . and you're wondering how I can help you get over the cravings . . . is that right so far . . .?*
- *Now that you've decided you want to cut out alcohol altogether there are several possibilities that we can discuss right now . . . and perhaps you've already been thinking along these lines . . . tell me your initial thoughts . . .*

Reflective listening then is an important skill to learn if you want to avoid the roadblocks that can stop people abruptly in their tracks. You can think of it as building a stable platform from which you can launch an effective change process. Without it you are simply treading water. You don't have to overdo it though. A few simple, well-timed statements may be all that is required to create a window of opportunity to make a real difference in someone's life – on their terms.

Chapter 6 outline summary
Major roadblocks

Roadblocks that get in the way of effective change consultations
- *Prescribing solutions*
- *Being judgmental*
- *Ignoring*
- *Cross-examining*

Respectful listening
- Attend to *non-verbal cues* (posture, gesture, breathing, eye gaze etc.)
- Use *minimal encouragers* as a signal to continue (ums and ahs etc.)
- Ask *open questions* for change (especially how and what)

Reflective listening
Accurately echoes back information, feelings, understandings and emotions
– using their own 'hot' words – ranges from superficial to deep
- *Content* –clarify and paraphrase information
- *Feelings* – underlying emotions about the issues under discussion
- *Intuitions* – check out your 'mind-reads' directly with the patient for accuracy
- *Summarising* – use their words to précis the narrative thus far
- *Signposting* – using information gathered to signal the next step

Kick 'but' . . . without 'try'ing

The word 'but' is an interesting one. The way people use it can tell you a lot about what is really going on for them. The way *you* use it can strengthen or weaken your persuasion message – but don't take my word for that. One of the most exasperating consultations you can get into is the 'yes, but' consultation. You probably recognise the scenario that goes along the lines of anything you suggest being met with that phrase.

I tried that but *it didn't work . . .*

The other doctor suggested that but *it didn't work either . . .*

My friend took that medication but *it didn't help her any . . .*

I really want to change this but *I don't have the willpower . . .*

I tried something like that last year but *it didn't do anything for me . . .*

I really want to do what you suggest but *I just can't . . .*

I like the look of that but *it doesn't feel right . . .*

I'll give it a go but *I don't think it'll work out . . .*

I agree with you but *. . .*

These kinds of consultations tend to go downhill rapidly and may end in impasse, with a frustrating silence. It is the kind of circumstance that often prevails when, as the clinician, you have been arguing for the benefits of change or pushing a particular line of action that you think will be beneficial. What is really going on here? Well, the word 'but' is a signal of incongruence. It has a tendency to negate anything that comes before it. The first half of the sentence says one thing whilst the second half says something altogether different.

We are all inclined to do this at some time or another. For some people, however, it can be a very habitual pattern. We can call them polarity responders – they will very often say and do the very opposite of what you say. They seem to carve out their very existence by describing themselves in terms of how they are different from everything and everybody else. They mark out the exceptions to everything you say. If they don't do this they may feel, at some level, as if they don't exist. Every interaction may feel like an argument. It is not personal – they're not deliberately trying to wind you up. This is simply how they communicate. On the whole, though, remember that none of us generally likes being told explicitly what we should do and may feel our hackles spontaneously rising even before we have considered the merits of any proposal.

You can also say 'but' non-verbally too. You don't have to utter the word for its unspoken influence to be apparent. Paying attention to a person's posture, gestures and voice tone as they are speaking will give a running commentary as to whether they are congruent – the words, tones and body language matching – or incongruent. This will give you lots of clues as to whether or not that particular person is likely to put their words into action.

Here are some examples where the 'but' is left unsaid:

Yes . . . I'll do that . . . (said with a sigh) . . .

Well if you're sure that's the right thing to do . . . (simultaneous shake of the head no) . . .

On the one hand what you're saying makes complete sense . . .

I want to . . . (wistful look into the distance) . . .

OK, I'll do that . . . (simultaneous grimace) . . .

No, there's nothing else . . . (eyes roving left and right) . . .

Of course I don't mind . . . (said with a sigh, looking away) . . .

I'm sure this will work out . . . (flat monotone, eyes down right) . . .

KICKING 'BUT'

There are several ways that you can deal with the kinds of communication scenarios that involve the word 'but'. It will help you enormously if you have already come to know your own internal signals for congruence and incongruence (*see* Chapter 5). You can use them as a barometer of the interaction. They will alert you to the nuances that are ever present, yet often unnoticed.

Firstly you can simply notice the verbal and non-verbal signals of 'but' and store them away for later use. You don't have to jump in immediately to challenge them. Sometimes it is more powerful to gather several examples of this communication pattern before reflecting it back to the person concerned. At times it may be more useful not to draw conscious attention to the pattern – simply use it back on them.

For those who are polarity responders or give you a series of 'yes, buts' you can change your own communication style to make it more likely that they will consider your information rather than dismiss it out of hand. Rather than giving a suggestion of what they can or should do, you tell them what they can't or shouldn't do instead . . . together with a strategic 'but' in the right direction. Here are some examples.

You probably won't believe this but . . .

You're possibly very unlikely to do this but . . .

This may not work for you either but . . .

You're probably not sure that this is the right thing for you but . . .

I have an idea that you may reject out of hand but . . .

If you think of the word 'but' as the fulcrum point around which two sentences balance then reversing the order can change the whole experience, sometimes very favourably. In other cases it can act as an intervention in its own right. More usually, though, it loosens the thinking around a problem area by subtly changing a habitual communication pattern. Notice the shift in your experience with the next example:

I'll do it . . . but . . . I'm not sure it'll work . . .

becomes

You're not sure it'll work . . . but . . . you'll do it . . .

I'll stay away from the pub on Friday . . . but . . . it will be difficult . . .

becomes

It will be difficult . . . but . . . you'll stay away from the pub on Friday . . .

Sometimes the 'but' is left unsaid, either with a pregnant pause or with an accompanying non-verbal message. There are several ways to deal with this. You can lean forward in your chair with a quizzical look and say 'but?' You can ask if they have any unspoken reservations. If you have developed your skills sufficiently you can play back both parts of the incongruence to them at the same time. Here are some examples:

But . . .? (with a quizzical look)

I'm curious . . . when you said you would do that . . . did you have some reservations?

I can't help thinking that at some level part of you doesn't agree with something I've said . . .?

You're certain you agree to that then . . .? (simultaneously shaking your head 'no')

You're absolutely correct . . . you probably won't find this easy (nodding your head 'yes' simultaneously).

Occasionally you may want to use the negation effect of 'but' on the previous sentence to get across a particular message in a useful way. You are then deliberately using it to imply the opposite of the original meaning. Some examples will help clarify.

Change may not be easy . . . but . . . when you learn the right steps anything is possible . . .

Mastering this material quickly may seem challenging . . . but . . . the benefits are life-changing . . .

You may not think you can readily assimilate the skills in this book effortlessly . . . but . . . how good will you feel when colleagues begin commenting on how you're using it all automatically . . .?

'AND'

Sometimes it can be very effective to substitute the word 'and' for 'but'. This has the effect of joining sentences, and therefore experiences, more seamlessly. Whereas 'but' can act as a stumbling block, 'and' tends to smooth over the joins. What's more, the consequence is that you can remain aligned with your communication partner, simultaneously seeing things from their point of view whilst leading them in a different direction. You maintain, and may even deepen, your rapport whilst opening up further possibilities for change. Try the following pairs of statements on for size and feel the difference between each.

> *I understand you're finding it difficult* but *I'd like you to consider the following . . .*

becomes

> *I understand you're finding it difficult* and *I'd like you to consider the following . . .*

> *I know you can do this* but *so far you haven't . . . what's stopping you . . .?*

becomes

> *I know you can do this* and *so far you haven't . . . what's stopping you . . .?*

> *I realise you are a resourceful person* but *this is a real challenge . . .*

becomes

> *I realise you are a resourceful person* and *this is a real challenge . . .*

You may already have noticed that certain framing words, when used at the start of your next sentence can foster even more agreement and rapport, especially when used in conjunction with 'and'. They let someone know that you have fully heard and taken on board what they have said, appreciating their circumstances and experiences and acknowledging the depth of their feelings. This acknowledgment can be a very powerful intervention in its own right. You can practise with the following words.

> *I understand, I appreciate, I recognise, I realise, I know, I respect, I agree, I identify with, I value, I admire, understandably, justifiably, reasonably . . . all with 'and' . . .*

But please don't do any of this unless you really want to get skilled at it. And don't even think that it's possible to learn how to, very quickly indeed. Some people hate writing out their own examples, but then they're not going to get as accomplished as someone who does. I appreciate it may seem less than easy and on the same hand, growing your expertise, bit by bit, can be so satisfying, can't it?

IT CAN BE SO 'TRY'ING . . .

The word 'try' is another one of those little words that can tell so much. And like 'but' you can find ways to use it more effectively too. Mostly, when someone says they will *try* to do something the underlying assumption is that of failure. Try can either signify that the person is very unlikely to attempt what they've said they'll do, or if they do, it will be a half-hearted effort that is unlikely to succeed. Consider the following statements from patients and notice how the results are almost a foregone conclusion:

> *I'll* try *to give up smoking next week . . .*

> *I'll* try *not to eat that bar of chocolate . . .*

> *I'll* try *to say 'no' to drugs . . .*

> *I'll* try *not to use my credit card this weekend . . .*

> *I'll* try *to put this into action as you suggest . . .*

As clinicians we often fall into the same trap when we give patients our suggestions for what we think they should do next. It can be very insidious.

> *I'd like you to* try *this medication and see how you get on . . .*

> *I suggest you* try *to do something different with your hands when you get the urge to smoke . . .*

> *Why don't you* try *to give up drinking . . .?*

> *It would really be in your best interests if you* try *to take more exercise, you know . . .*

> Try *to put less food on your plate . . .*

So rather than asking people to try to do something, what can you do instead? The simplest thing to do is to either ask a direct question or make a statement that uses the words 'can' and 'will'. This is a tester of their current degree of commitment. You can also soften this a bit to take the hard edge off. One of the benefits of so doing is that you will be able to read their non-verbal response just before or simultaneously with their verbal one. This will give you more information about whether they are likely to follow through or not. Using some of the same examples as above, notice how different it is to be on the receiving end.

Will you take this medication for two weeks and let me know the results . . .?

When you get the urge to smoke you can do something different with your hands . . .

Can I ask you a question . . .? When will you consider giving up drinking . . .?

Taking more exercise is important . . . can you commit to that . . .?

I'm curious to know whether you can put less food on your plate . . .?

Initially you might be forgiven for thinking that we should try to eliminate the word 'try' altogether. Rather than getting rid of it completely we can find a particular niche where it can be very useful. This is the time when you actually want someone to succeed in failing. This may sound confusing at first because usually we want to point people clearly in the direction of success. The following examples, used after a successful therapeutic intervention, will shed some light and show you how to do this.

I want you to try in vain to have that problem you used to have . . .

Try hard to go back to the old ways and notice what happens . . .

You can always try hard not to succeed in continuing to be a nonsmoker . . .

Try as hard as you can to fight off the overwhelming urge to exercise . . .

This little interlude has been all about how to kick 'buts' without 'try'ing. In the persuasion process these two words are vital to master. My question is: Will you commit to putting what you have learned into daily practice? You can always try just hard enough to succeed at failing not to use this in every consultation. You may have found that last sentence a bit confusing, but please don't pay attention to anything other than doing the very best you can to help people change easily and successfully. Anything less than fully mastering persuasion in practice just won't get the results you deserve.

Interlude 1 outline summary

'But'
- Has a tendency to separate and negate whatever comes before it in a sentence
- Can often be a signal for incongruency
- Can be 'said' non-verbally (voice tone, posture, gesture, eye movements)
- Can be used repetitively as a polarity response (Yes . . . but)

Kicking 'but'
Strategies in consultations
- Notice it but don't mention it
- Gather several examples then discuss at a process level
- If 'but' is the fulcrum point for two sentences, then reverse them
- Reflect back both sides of the incongruency verbally and non-verbally
- Use 'but' deliberately for polarity responders . . . 'You won't believe this . . . but'
- Use it to get your message across . . . 'Changing may not be easy . . . but . . . when you learn the right steps anything is possible . . .'

'And'
- Can often be used in place of 'but'
- Joins unrelated experiences together
- Even more effective when used after . . . 'I understand, I appreciate, I recognise, I realise, I know . . . and . . .'

'Try'
- Underlying assumption of half-hearted attempt or failure
- Lack of commitment to task
- Use in reverse . . . 'Try hard not to give in to the urge to exercise . . .'

Raising awareness

Many people who turn up on our doorsteps are unaware that they have a problem brewing. They may be immersed in a sea of denial that their current behaviours are injurious to their long-term health. Perhaps they turn up because external circumstances have forced them against their will (e.g. spouse, children, boss). They are really not invested in making any changes on their own behalf and may simply pay lip service to any advice offered.

This group tend to be very short on information about their problem, even if they know they have one in the first place. They generally don't discuss their behavioural patterns and may become highly defensive if challenged. They tend to avoid learning about who and what have really created their symptoms. What's more, they do not pay any attention to future consequences and even if they did they are unlikely to take personal responsibility for them.

Some may have abandoned themselves to the belief that nothing can change now. They may even claim that they have tried everything and nothing has ever worked for them. The sad thing about them is that they may well be doomed unless they are helped – but we are often doomed ourselves because we offer help in the wrong way. Sometimes life transitions can pave the way for change (becoming a parent, grandparent, reaching the big '4-0'). Occasionally social pressures can assist (no-smoking zones, for example). Yet in the main, the maxim 'ignorance is bliss' prevails.

Make no mistake about it though. Diseases such as ischaemic heart disease, diabetes and cancer are partly related to lifestyle choices. Childhood obesity is on a marked exponential increase. Many people are walking blindly into dysfunction, disease and even death. As clinicians we need to find ways to intervene in a manner that can respect everyone's choices.

We need to ask ourselves a fundamental question:

What is the positive intention that underlies this stage?

The answer is *safety*. This is a feeling that pervades this stage, the feeling of being safe, secure and comfortable. Any change is viewed as being 'un-safe', 'in-secure' and 'un-comfortable'. Many people vastly overestimate the costs and markedly underestimate the benefits of changing.

We can sort this group out into four general categories or subgroups: reluctant, rebellious, resigned and rationalising. Below are both descriptions and some strategies for dealing with each.

Reluctant

People who are reluctant to change usually do so from a base of lack of knowledge combined with inertia. They are not fully conscious of the effects of their problem or current situation. They may feel relatively safe and comfortable where they are, mainly because they are fearful of change. In motivation terms, they move *away from* the pain of the unknown.

It is often very important with this subgroup to allow them to explore their reluctance in a non-judgmental, non-threatening way, without pushing too hard initially. The following questions are very useful:

> *What concerns do you have about making changes?*

> *Could there be any positives about changing?*

> *How much worse would your current situation need to get before you considered changing?*

The third question can prove very helpful here. It uses their own strategy of moving away from pain and turns it back on the present problem. This can provide an initial 'push' that moves them towards changing. It fits with a more general plan of making the status quo uncomfortable and change more comfortable.

ROGER

Roger was a 52-year-old recently diagnosed with Type 2 diabetes. Some 25 kg overweight he enjoyed a sedentary lifestyle which included several business lunches a week. His weight had gradually ballooned over the previous decade almost with his recognising it. He enjoyed rich food and wine, saw himself as a gourmand and was initially reluctant to think about making changes. He was particularly concerned about what his business colleagues might think if he were to start eating 'all that rabbit food'.

Initially he couldn't see any positives about changing, though he became more interested when the dietician showed him some information on how to cook exotic dishes that were diabetic-friendly. Perhaps some of the local restaurants that he went to on a regular basis might incorporate some dishes specifically for him. He really didn't want to change but when he could also foresee that his additional risk of ischaemic heart disease might lead to angina – or worse, death from a heart attack, like his father – he found himself with much food for thought.

Rebellious

People who are rebellious are usually heavily invested in what they are currently doing. They may be very hostile and resistant, expressing themselves and their views in no uncertain terms and manner. If you engage in arguing with them you may well meet your match . . . and more. Their unspoken rule is: *No one tells me what to do.* They will give you a barrow-load of reasons as to why they are not going to change and may be actually quite knowledgeable about their problem behaviour.

It is often best to consider this person a polarity responder – someone who will do the opposite of whatever you say. They have a strong internal locus of control and have lots of energy. In these circumstances you have to frame your questions carefully. It's generally best to start out agreeing with them . . . then add a little twist.

> *You're right, you're probably not the kind of person who could . . . (X) . . . (stop smoking, start exercising etc.) . . . Or are you?*

> *Only you can decide if . . . (X) . . . makes sense to you . . . or not . . .*

This kind of language fits with their preferred patterns and makes it less easy for them to argue with you. Rebellious people make up their own minds firmly about change and when they do decide to change, their highly energised style often makes them determined to succeed. Psychologists call this phenomenon an extinction burst. From being argumentatively completely against a course of action they become its chief protagonist.

RACHEL

Rachel was an inveterate smoker of 40+ cigarettes a day. She said: 'I hope you're not one of those doctors who are going to harp on about stopping smoking . . . I can't stand that.'

I assured her I wasn't. In fact I agreed that she was probably very unlikely to be the kind of person who could stop easily and I could see from how she presented herself that no one was going to tell her what to do. In fact, given that she was looking a little stressed maybe she needed to smoke a little more!

She laughed and said: 'Well I'm not as bad as all that . . . and I could cut back if I really wanted to.' I told her I appreciated what she said and that only she could decide when she was ready to do so . . . though I did remark on the flying pig hovering just outside the consulting room window . . . then we went on to other things. Yet, several months later she asked me for some self-help literature on stopping smoking 'Just in case I'm ever tempted . . .' To which I replied 'Very unlikely . . .'

Resigned

People who are resigned have generally tried and failed to change several times and have no energy left. They feel completely overwhelmed at the prospect of change and may have given up hope. They may feel totally controlled by their habit. Their behaviour says: *it's too late for me . . .*

Sometimes it can be useful to let this group know that behavioural change may require several attempts before complete success occurs. Smokers have on average had four attempts to stop before finally succeeding. Despite these positive tales, however, they may remain very demoralised.

The most productive strategies here are to explore barriers to change and keep instilling hope that change can occur. This is one group in which the clinician's beliefs about change can become self-fulfilling prophecies. Because these patients are often so overwhelmed when thinking about change it may be very important to focus on taking tiny steps with achievable tasks to give a much-needed feeling of success (cut down by one cigarette in the day and so on.). Ask:

What obstacles get in the way of your changing . . .?

What one very small step could you think about taking . . .?

Lack of energy due to overwhelm is a key culprit preventing change. Using your chunking down skills to pinpoint one small yet attainable goal can help harness what little energy is available. Yet even a very small success can give a disproportionate energy boost.

RHONA

Rhona was a single parent of two under-10 children. She was also very overweight. Although she didn't eat very much during the day she found that, once she'd got the kids to bed, she literally pigged out on sweets, crisps and chocolate. She had tried so many different diets and come unstuck that she was resigned to remaining obese and felt herself unattractive.

The kids' going to bed was the signal for 'me time'. She felt stressed and down during the day and eating was the one thing that made her feel better, even though it was a temporary fix. She was too tired to do anything else with her time that late at night.

Rather than figure out yet another doomed-to-failure, late-night strategy to get her to stop overeating, another approach was called for. She and a friend contemplated signing up for a weekly salsa class. They would each go on alternate weeks and look after each other's kids. Then, on another night of the week, they would take turns to have everyone over to the same house and practise their steps.

Rationalising

Rationalisers have all the answers. They tend to intellectualise a lot and mini-mise any potential harm. They may know a great deal about their particular habit and can tell you why they especially are at less risk than someone else. They may say things like: *My grandfather smoked 60 cigarettes a day until he was age 90*. They have an internal locus of control but unlike the rebellious group they tend to remain in their heads rather than in their emotions.

The best strategies to use here are to explore all the possible benefits of their problem behaviour first before moving on to any potential negative aspects. If you try to beat them over the head with any negatives they come up with you will quickly lose rapport and they will become more entrenched. One of the best times to prod this group into action is if you catch them when they are more emotional or unwell as a result of their behaviour. Good questions are:

So what are all the positives about X (smoking, drinking, eating etc.) . . .?

Are there any negatives . . .?

Of course, only you can come to your own conclusions about changing . . . can't you?

It is vital that you do agree with all the positives they come up with rather than arguing with them. If you keep chunking up the benefits you will unearth the positive intention behind the problem. You can do this by asking iteratively: *and what's important about that?* Then you can speculate on how they could access the benefits using other behaviours. For example, if a benefit of smoking is relaxa-tion, what other behaviours could give the same result?

ROBERT

Robert was an unemployed, middle-aged binge drinker. He lacked social confidence and found that alcohol made him feel 'ten feet tall'. Rather than being concerned about his developing alcohol tolerance he rationalised that he was simply one of those people who could drink a lot without it affecting

him. Whenever his drinking was raised he would generally say: 'A big mus-
cled man like me can hold far more beer than a smaller guy.'

When his liver function tests became deranged he countered with: 'It's
only a number, Doc . . . I bet many people have had higher readings . . .
anyway I feel fine in myself . . . not like one of my drinking buddies who
really does look the worse for wear.' He really couldn't see any negatives for
himself even though they might happen to other people.

When he was arrested for a drink-driving offence that involved nar-
rowly missing a pensioner on a zebra crossing he came face to face with
his problem. He had never seen himself as a criminal and felt ashamed not
only for himself but also for his family. He couldn't rationalise this one away.
For the first time he opened up to the possibility that his drinking was doing
more damage than he'd originally thought . . . and perhaps he should do
something about it.

GOALS AND STRATEGIES FOR THIS STAGE

This stage is definitely *not* about getting people to take precipitate action. That
is a task that is not only very premature, it is almost certainly doomed to failure. The more your actions are perceived as a push to make a change now, the
more likely you will preserve the status quo. So just what are our aims for this
stage?

Most people at this juncture either do not know they have a potential problem – they are sailing along blissfully ignorant of the submerged hazards – or
are good at the various skills involved in denial or justification of their current
position. The main goal in any one stage is to do what is necessary to nudge
people into the next – no more, no less. Given that the next stage is resolving
ambivalence then our main task must be to *create ambivalence* in the first place.
This is our marker of success.

If ambivalence reflects being in two minds about something (e.g. whether
to stop smoking or not) then we need to generate a potential conflict to stew
over. We must tactfully stir up some incongruency and inconsistency between
values and behaviour. We must get them disturbed. In fact we could sum this
up by saying that if necessary:

> We must create a problem to move away from.

Of course it is important to be careful about how we do this. One very good
strategy is simply to give the awareness-raising information in a straightforward
manner as if you were discussing the weather, then turn to other matters in the
consultation without further ado. It may help to say:

Here is some information you might find useful . . . of course only you can decide what use you make of it . . .

Sometimes I have said in a jocular tone, rubbing my hands gleefully together:

If you carry on like this you'll be keeping me in business for a while yet . . . if you don't drop down dead first of course!

Occasionally, in a more serious tone if they have children I might say:

Do you want to survive to see your children grow up . . . or look into the eyes of your first grandchild?

If they are more of a polarity responder:

You're probably very unlikely to think carefully about the potential harm . . . or are you?

You're probably not going to believe me when I say . . . (harmful effects of condition).

Usually this is just about as far as you should take it as you remember the adage *less is more* for this stage. Occasionally some people who are on the verge of moving to the next stage would benefit from a specific task that raises their awareness of the problem habit (smoking, drinking, eating, gambling, addictions etc.). They may agree to keep a diary of the specific behaviour for a two-week period. This is not so that they focus on making changes, but simply to become more conscious of the habit itself and how it affects other areas of life that they haven't yet paid attention to. This however is a task more suited to the next stage.

Rather than being deadly serious, be a bit lighter-hearted in your approach instead. All you need to do is sow some seeds. The fruits may occur well in the future.

Chapter 7 outline summary

Raising awareness

There are four subgroups in this stage. Our task is to begin to raise just enough awareness to nudge them to the next stage.

Reluctant

- Fearful of change
- Move away from the unknown
- Lack of knowledge combined with inertia

Ask: *How much worse would your current situation need to get before you considered changing?*

Rebellious

- Heavily invested in current behaviours
- Hostile and resistant
- 'No one tells me what to do'

Ask: *You're right, you're probably not the kind of person who could easily stop . . . (smoking/drinking/overeating etc.) . . . or are you?*

Resigned

- Tried and failed several times
- Feel overwhelmed at the thought of changing
- Have run out energy

Ask: *What one very small step could you think about taking . . .?*

Rationalising

- Have all the answers
- Minimise potential harm of problem behaviours
- Remain 'in their heads', intellectualising

Ask: *What are all the positive benefits your current behaviour gives you . . .?*

Overall goals for this stage

- Create ambivalence
- Create a problem to move away from

Changing frames

The meaning we give to any behaviour depends entirely on how we frame it. A frame is the boundary that we put round an experience so that we can we make sense of it. A problem drinker may frame drinking alcohol as an enjoyable social event with friends. His spouse may view it as a nightmare of antisocial behaviour. It is the same event seen through different eyes with a different meaning.

Our habitual frames are long-term friends – so long-term that they infuse our whole being. We have lived with them day in, day out over such an extensive timeframe that we are no longer able to differentiate them. They are like a pair of spectacles; they change how we experience the world – and we forget we are wearing them. We assume that our frames represent the 'truth' of our current existence. We often fail to realise that they are only one way to interpret the world – amongst many others.

Our frames (beliefs, values, attitudes etc.) permeate our entire neurology. They are like a default mode, which is set to respond in a typical fashion, over and over again. Depression is a case in point. Not only do long-term sufferers see their world through the frames of negative automatic thoughts, their very bodily biochemistry (cortisol levels, etc.) is adversely affected too. In a sense, frames not only have a signature thinking style, they also give rise to a signature physiology and to signature behaviours.

Frames tend to have an all-or-nothing quality to them. They are a bit like a light switch – either on or off. Our main aim as clinicians is help people switch to frames that are more useful for their particular circumstances. It is a bit like giving them a different set of spectacles to look through. The world may initially appear very different, even confusing, until they become accustomed to seeing things in this new light.

Changing frames (or re-framing) is an approach that accepts the 'truth' of a person's current way of assimilating the raw data of experience and offers a new meaning or interpretation for them to try on instead. We help them see the old habitual experience in a new light, which can assist them in moving towards the kinds of change they want to make. When done well this can literally be life-changing.

There are three general categories of changing frames. We can 're-frame', 'out-frame' and 'de-frame' the problems people offer to us. Re-framing is changing the meaning of the original problem behaviour or finding another context in which it is more useful. Outframing is enlarging the scope of the current problem situation by enveloping it in a bigger framework which has more positive connotations. De-framing is breaking the problem issue into smaller component parts and dealing with them piecemeal.

In the next section we will take examples of common clinical presentations and use various changing-frames patterns to offer new meanings and interpretations.

PATTERNS OF CHANGING FRAMES

Changing frames is not a 'one step and you're free' type of intervention. It is simply a way to help someone get a different perspective on a problem situation. You can think of it as loosening the glue that holds a problem together. Sometimes the solvent works surprisingly quickly. At others it is just one of a multitude of things you are bringing to bear to help change occur. You will also find that all of the patterns below can also be used to successfully defuse resistance behaviour too.

In the sections that follow we will see the effect of various patterns on some common clinical scenarios. Here are three typical presentations in day-to-day practice. We will use them as examples for each of the patterns. Notice the shifts that the new thinking can make.

1   I can't stop eating when I feel down.
2   Coming off drugs is very difficult.
3   My heart is too damaged to take exercise.

Redefining

When you redefine you simply take one or more of the words in the original statement and substitute others. The new words can begin to modify the original meaning and begin to lead towards change. Whenever someone gives you a statement like this, ask yourself:

What else could this mean . . .?

1   So you can't stop putting certain things in your mouth when you don't feel so good inside.

2   You feel that stopping certain medications can be more challenging than others.

3   Your heart muscle isn't yet at the stage where you can increase your daily activities.

Remember, all we are looking for here is a small acceptable change in the meaning, which you can build on later. You simply want to 'loosen the glue'.

Consequence

Every frame has its consequences, both positive and negative. By taking the current frame out into the future you can make the costs of remaining the same seem very stark. If they don't change now, this is what they might have to look forward to. A useful question to ask yourself is:

What will happen if they continue in this way . . .?

1   What will happen if you get so big you can't get up?

2   How much more difficult will it be to stop if you continue like this for another five years?

3   How much weaker might your heart muscle get if you remain less active?

Prior intention

All behaviours, even negative ones, are trying to do something of importance for us. There is an underlying positive purpose which, when unearthed, can sow the seeds of change. Ask yourself:

What is this behaviour doing for them . . .?

1   Currently, eating is the one thing that helps you *feel good* . . . at least for a while . . . until you find other ways to get the same effect long term . . .

2   That's right, it's because the challenge is how to get the *positive things* drugs give you in a much healthier way.

3   What we need to do is to plan how to *safely and securely* rebuild your heart muscle using workouts you can do easily.

Counterexample

Because frames appear as all-or-nothing phenomena, then one good counterexample can help make a significant shift. It is generally more useful to help people find a counterexample in their own experience. They can more easily discount one that you give from your own. Ask yourself:

What are the exceptions to their current frame . . .?

1 Have you ever had a time when you felt down but did something different instead of eating?
2 Have you ever had a time when you stopped drugs even for a short time?
3 Do you know anyone who had a previously damaged heart yet now exercises freely?

You can use the answers to these exceptional times to find out just how the counterexample happened, what part they had to play in it and how they could use the same skills to make this happen again.

Apply back to itself

This is where you take the statement that someone makes and apply the same logic to it recursively. You can also use the same words back on themselves. This may appear to be counterintuitive, yet it can be surprising how quickly you can loosen a limiting frame. This is one where you simply reflexively give the reframe on the spur of the moment.

1 It eats you up inside when you're down on yourself.
   Oh no . . . so you'll starve yourself when you feel really good?
2 You're right, maybe you need a drug to help you get off drugs.
   Is that a drug-induced statement?
3 So, your heart's not really in it then?
   Exercising your mind in that way will damage your heart further.

These kinds of spontaneous reframes can provoke anything from mild confusion to bursts of laughter. They are the kinds of states that are very useful in any change process. By interrupting the problem frame they open people up to the possibility of considering other perspectives.

Another outcome

What you are saying here is that the current issue is not really the relevant one – it's something completely different instead. You can use this to help focus people on a new result to aim for. Ask yourself:

What is another outcome to focus on . . .?

1 The real issue is not your eating . . . it's about what other choices you can make to take care of your deeper needs in a more effective way.
2 Perhaps it isn't about whether or not it's difficult . . . maybe it's about what you are going to do instead with all your free time once you've kicked the habit.

3   Possibly the first exercise is to rebuild your self-confidence.

Chunking down

In this category you take one element of the frame and focus down on it, getting much more specific. This is like getting to the individual tree of what seemed like a veritable, overwhelming forest. In so doing you can make what initially seems like a small change which then resonates throughout the whole, changing the frame altogether. Ask yourself:

What are examples or parts of this . . .?

1   What things specifically do you eat?
    Give me an example of what gets you down.
2   Which drug specifically is more difficult to get off?
    Is it deciding to stop using the drug, the withdrawal symptoms or staying off altogether over time that is more challenging?
3   Do you know how much of your heart has been damaged and how much is healthy?
    What specific types of exercise are you thinking about?

Often people's frames are couched in abstract or global terms. You can use the more detailed answers from these questions to generate solutions for change that the person may not have thought of previously.

Chunking up

In this category you are taking a specific element of the frame and generalising it – making it more abstract or global. Firstly find out what is important to them in the situation. Then find which bigger, higher-level category it fits into. It often helps to playfully exaggerate this by taking it to the limit. Ask yourself:

What's important here . . .? What is this an example of . . .? How can I exaggerate this and take it to the limit . . .?

1   If you get mega-depressed then you may well get so big you'll explode!
2   Withdrawal methods are not reliable for contraception either!
3   I hope you don't go 'twang' when someone pulls at your emotional heartstrings!

You may need plenty of rapport with the individual before you use these playful exaggerations. Ensure you have a smile on your face and a twinkle in your eye when using them.

Hierarchy of criteria

Criteria are the particular values that are important to someone in a specific situation. Because some values are more important than others we can use them to leverage the lesser ones to good effect. Simply ask yourself:

What is more important than this . . .?

1   When you learn some simple skills that can improve your confidence and self-esteem your binge eating will no longer be an issue.
2   What's more important . . . focusing on the difficulties of getting off drugs . . . or feeling the deep pleasure of being really free at last?
3   Perhaps strengthening your remaining healthy heart muscle will help you spend more quality time with your grandchildren.

Changing frame size

In this category you can change frames by looking at time (longer or shorter frames), people (larger or smaller numbers), and perspectives (the bigger or smaller picture). One useful way to do this is to ask about universal experiences by using the following words:

All? Every? Always? Never? Timeframes?

1   So when people feel down they always eat for relief?
    What did you do in the past before you used food as a comfort?
2   So everybody always finds coming off all drugs difficult?
    Have you ever stayed off for five minutes? An hour? A day? A week?
3   Will that always be the case in the future as it strengthens without your noticing?
    You may well be amazed at what three months of cardiac rehabilitation can do.

Meta-frame

A meta-frame establishes a frame *about* a frame. It's a bit like having a helicopter view of the situation. From this perspective you can reflect on the thoughts, beliefs, feelings and behaviours that make up the frame and evaluate it by giving a different interpretation or meaning. The question to ask yourself is:

How is it possible they could believe this . . .?

1   You only believe this because you haven't yet been able to change your state by other equally accessible means.
2   You only believe this because you haven't yet met people who have

actually come off drugs and stayed off them.

3 You only believe this because you don't know how strongly heart muscle can adapt with the right stimulus.

Because you are challenging a deeply held belief you may want to use some softeners (*I'm wondering whether . . . I'm curious if . . . etc.*) to make the statements appear less confrontational.

Other people

In this category we can check to see if this frame holds true in other people's experience. If our frames are simply one way of experiencing the world then how would someone else, with a completely different set of frames, think and behave differently. Ask yourself:

Who would see it differently . . .?

1 Some people believe that if you sort out *what's eating you* then you'll feel much better more of the time.
2 One of my patients who came off drugs said that his main difficulty was actually getting out of the circle of 'friends' that had kept him in his habit.
3 Let me introduce you to some patients who have gone through our cardiac rehab programme who can tell you first-hand how much more they're able to do in their lives.

Discriminatory strategy

The way we represent our frames to ourselves is often out of conscious awareness. We may be unable not only to differentiate the frame we are using in our current situation but also to discriminate why we use this one rather than another. By bringing this into awareness we get a chance to access and update our frames accordingly. Ask yourself:

How specifically do they know this is true/not true . . .?

1 How do you know if it's true that eating helps when you feel down?
  How would you know if the reverse actually happened instead?
2 How do you represent in your mind's eye that getting off drugs is difficult?
  How would you know if it were easier than you think?
3 How do you know if it's true that your heart is too damaged?
  How would you know if it were actually stronger than you think it is?

You can use any of these changing frames patterns at all stages of the persuasion-in-practice process. Rather than having to remember the specific patterns by name you can refer to the questions template below for easy reference.

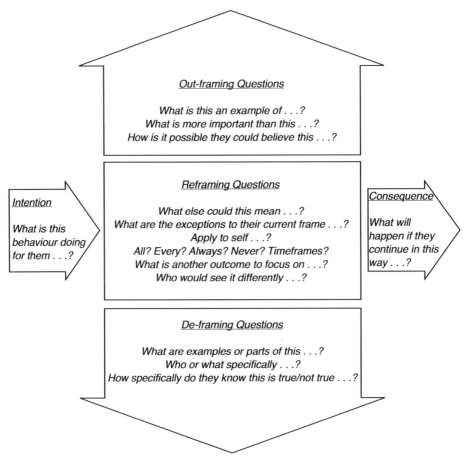

FIGURE A Changing frames questions

Resolving ambivalence

This is the stage where people acknowledge that they do indeed have a problem and begin to contemplate doing something about it. However, thinking about it and actually doing something about it are two entirely different things. Ambivalence is an inner polarity response whereby people ruminate between the two poles of the change argument. In effect they are saying *I want to change and I don't want to change* . . . at the same time. This can be a very confusing state to be in and some people may go round in ruminative circles with an increasing feeling of exasperation and frustration. In fact some chronic contemplators who have remained stuck in this feeling for months or even years may become quite depressed.

Sometimes 'stuckness' results from wishful thinking. This is when you want things to be different without having to do anything uncomfortable to make the change happen. You want all the benefits of remaining the same . . . plus the change of course. For some people the talk is all about the changes they are going to make when the time is right. However, when pressed, the time is never right. Change can be quite scary – it's all about dealing with uncertainty. Many of us want to be completely certain things will work out in advance prior to taking the first step . . . and no one can guarantee that.

As clinicians we may have a strong urge to step in, resolve the ambivalence and get patients to commit to action. Resist it! If you don't, you are likely to do more harm than good. The rush to premature commitment usually leaves casualties along the way, the main one being the patient's change process. In truth we often need to *increase* the ambivalence even more and explore each side of it skilfully and thoroughly before resolution can take place. And even then, resolution does not necessarily mean action.

Sometimes patients may have already decided their goals and outcomes and may even know the steps they can take to get there. However, they may not be *ready to change*. Others are thinking about changing in a more intellectual and dissociated way. They have not yet personalised the relevant information to their own symptoms and behaviours. They may know in general what can happen to long-term smokers and drinkers – they haven't yet stepped fully into the picture themselves. They require specific, accurate, personal feedback about their habits (perhaps blood tests such as cholesterol levels, liver function tests or lung function tests). For some, though not all, this can provide powerful feedback.

For effective change to occur it is vital to acknowledge the positive function played by the problem behaviour. We are often perplexed as clinicians when, despite all the acknowledged mounting negatives, our patients persist in engaging in another drink, another cigarette, another chocolate cake, spending sprees at the shops, more illicit drugs, sitting on the couch watching more television, etc. The answer is really quite simple. The momentary benefit and surge of good feelings in the here and now that they get from these behaviours currently outweighs both the future benefits of changing and the pain they think it will cost them to get there. It is imperative that we recognise and explore these issues in depth.

QUESTIONS ARE THE ANSWER!

Before we can resolve ambivalence we must find out what lies at its heart. This means exploring both the pros and cons of changing . . . and of *not* changing. This does not have to be an exhaustive, all-encompassing search, but it does need to cover all the quadrants below. Failing to adequately traverse all these parameters will likely lead to premature action and early relapse. Unasked fundamental questions will come back to haunt you.

Change is an emotional process. If it were merely rational then people could change what they want, whenever they wanted, simply by thinking about it intellectually. Of course we know that rarely happens (unless you are a relative of *Star Trek's* Mr Spock). Emotions light the spark of the change flame. Naturally, fire can burn painfully if we're not careful – we'd better not get too close. It can also light the way ahead and act as a beacon that attracts us.

In a similar way, emotional feelings give the energetic push and pull that would otherwise leave change ungrounded, in the academic realm only. We push away from pain and move towards the pleasure of getting what we want. If you are not achieving your goals it is because you are attaching more pain to

Benefits of changing	Benefits of current problem
Costs of not changing	Obstacles to changing

FIGURE 8.1 Costs and benefits of changing

getting there than pleasure. We need to harness and sequence this energy and put it to work – effectively. Reason and emotion need to work together synergistically. The following questions will show you how.

COSTS OF NOT CHANGING

We are going to start with the costs of *not* changing. This is because for many people, unless they are faced with the stark consequences of continuing their current behaviour, they may well fail to kick-start the change process. The basic question is:

What will it cost you in the future if you don't change now?

It is really important to get people to develop a sensory-rich picture of all the costs – both for them personally and their loved ones. They need to vividly imagine, in detail, the negative images that will sensitise them to the drawbacks of their behaviour. For the smoker, perhaps it would be the rasping wheeze of tortured lungs and the copious expectorated green phlegm, together with the tight, breathless feeling on minimal activity; for the binge eater, the massively ballooning weight, arthritic knees and hips and the red, malodorous rash of intertrigo. You need to encourage them to come up with their own personal believable imagery rather than impose your own.

Effects on family, friends and loved ones are important to include. Although, on the face of it, it may seem very harsh, I do encourage smokers with young children to imagine what the effect of their demise would be on them. Even to the extent of funeral arrangements and wailing children's voices. This has been particularly effective as a major spur to commit to action for many males. Here are some other questions you can use.

Box 8.1 Costs of not changing

What do you think will happen if you don't change anything?
What do you imagine are the worst things that might happen to you?
How has this problem stopped you from doing what you want in life?
If you do nothing at all, how bad do you think things will get?
What is the ultimate price you will pay if you don't change now?

RHONA'S COSTS

Rhona was already unhappy about her weight. She could see things spiralling out of control if she didn't act now. She saw herself with rolls of fat around her ankles. She felt even more unattractive and thought the possibilities of her having another relationship were receding into the distance. She could see how she'd already restricted her social life, using the kids as an excuse for her lack of confidence. She imagined what might happen when the kids eventually left home – the thought of being all on her own was enough to make her think about reaching for the crisps again.

BENEFITS OF CHANGING

Most advertisers know that they need to create the right image for their product to make it very attractive to their targeted selling group. They want to stir up thoughts and emotions that merge with the striking images to create a desire that pulls people into buying mode. We need to do the same thing in persuading someone to change behaviour. We need to get them to create a self-image that they yearn to have and which compels them to think and act in health-sustaining ways. The basic question is:

What would be the greatest benefits of making this change now?

Once again it is important to build a sensory-rich picture of just how different things would be for them, having made the change. For the smoker, they might picture healthy lungs, a strongly beating heart, and the physical energy that comes from feeling fit and healthy (plus a sackful of cash). For the binge eater you could ask them to imagine in detail how they would walk, talk, breathe and move, dressed in great looking clothes at their target weight. Really get them to step inside these scenarios and literally try them on for size. Encourage them to feel as if they're living the experience. Remember that emotional juice counts, so juice it up.

Keep in mind the positive effects of making the change on family, friends, colleagues and loved ones. Get them to think of themselves as role models. Ask them what their spouse, children (or grandchildren) might say when they've achieved their goal and get them to feel that resultant feeling deep within their heart. You really do want them to have a 'heartfelt' experience of a very positive kind. Think of yourself as a great state-inducer – the more intense the positive state the greater the attraction. Here are some more questions you can use.

Box 8.2 Benefits of changing

How would you be like as a person if things were really different?
What might be the best results you could imagine?
What would your life be like in five years if you really changed now?
Having made the change, what would improve the most?

ROBERT'S BENEFITS

Binge-drinking Robert had already begun to count the costs after his arrest. However, he wasn't really very clear initially on the benefits of long-term sobriety. With some prompting he recognised that he would be a very different person indeed, almost alien to his present self. Gradually it dawned on him that in many respects he would be like he was some 15 years previously – leaner, certainly fitter than his current standing and with a lot more money in his pocket. He liked the thought of that. His relationship with his wife would certainly change – he wasn't entirely sure if this would be for the better or not!

CONNECTING TO WHAT'S REALLY IMPORTANT

One area of vital importance is to chunk up on the perceived benefits of changing so as to connect with deeply held, core values. This is often called *laddering*, where the answer to one question is stepped up the rungs of an imaginary ladder to generate even more meaningful significance. When you touch these deeper values it can unleash a very powerful mechanism for change. You can take the answers to the previous sets of questions and leverage them in the following way until there comes a point when they simply don't have a more significant answer to give.

> *And what's really important to you about that?*

You can ask this question iteratively of each answer by saying:

> *And in achieving that, what would that do for you that is even more important?*

And finally:

> *So ultimately, what would this really mean to you?*

For Rhona our binge eater above who, on thinking about the benefits of changing had visualised herself looking great at her target weight, the answers to all three questions were:

> *My kids would say I looked fantastic.*

> *My confidence would soar.*

> *For the first time in my life I'd feel free to be me!*

Finding out about yourself in this way can be both immensely satisfying and give you a profound sense of connection to what really matters in your life. It can act as a wellspring of motivational power that can help you make the changes that you want. It lays bare your previously hidden deepest inner drives.

Box 8.3 Other useful laddering questions

And what purpose does this serve for you?

Imagine for a moment you achieved all that . . . what does that get for you?

Ultimately, what does this really mean about you . . . the kind of person you truly are?

BENEFITS OF CURRENT PROBLEM

Most people consider problems as things to be got rid of at the earliest opportunity. It's as if they are the less savoury parts of ourselves that pop out when least expected or wanted. No matter how much we try to 'will them away' they don't appear to be under conscious control. We judge ourselves harshly, feel deeply embarrassed and may want to kill off these aspects so they never return. Unfortunately this often makes the situation worse rather than better.

Some people, on the other hand, like their problems and are loathe to give them up. They make excuses for them, defend them, and may attack others who suggest they change. This is more common in the previous stage but can occur here too.

It is often useful to think of problem behaviours as our best attempts to achieve something of value for us. They are often our strategy, our way of relieving negative feelings that we don't wish to have. For example, many people who overeat may have some or many of the following issues: fear of deprivation, abandonment, loss, feelings of loneliness and emptiness, and negative feelings such as anxiety, guilt, fear and anger.

Engaging in risky behaviours – especially drugs and the surrounding culture – can give people not only a sense of connection and aliveness but also purpose and meaning to life, even if it kills them. Sometimes these risky behaviours can be used to get back at someone in a co-dependent type of relationship. At other times, activities such as smoking may help someone cope with a difficult partner or kids.

Our problem behaviours help us to escape from difficult situations and cope with challenging feelings – anger, fear, unresolved grief, depression, overwhelm, inadequacy, even unwanted intimacy. They are often our best way in the moment of helping us feel safe, secure, protected, loved and cared for. They may give us short-term pleasure to escape the everyday pains of living. We frequently use them to generate feelings of confidence, courage, power and even bliss. We can unearth similar sorts of feelings and emotions in drinkers, gamblers, smokers, drug addicts, couch potatoes etc. In short we often use our problems to help *change our state*.

So, it often very helpful to think that what we label as 'problem behaviour' is our current best response we can make in the situation. We can assume we have good reasons for behaving the way we do even though initially we might scratch our heads wondering what they may be. We need to become curious about the potential underlying message which has up until now remained unheard. Assuming that this negative aspect has a valued contribution to make can allow us to become less judgmental and more curious.

After setting this way of thinking as a framework with your patient you can ask:

> *What positive things might this problem actually be doing for you?*

You can take each answer through the laddering process until you find an important value that underlies the problem issue. For Rhona, our binge eater who periodically gorged, the answers were:

> *It stops me feeling lonely and empty.*

> *It makes me feel good inside.*

> *It's the one thing I do for myself.*

> *In those moments I feel totally loved and cared for.*

Rhona equated food with a strong sense of being loved. No wonder it had been such a difficult habit to break. This was one of the very few ways, perhaps the only way, that she could have access to these very powerful feelings. And of course this was something she could access for herself whenever she wanted. Unfortunately though, these feelings were short-lived and were replaced by self-loathing and disgust, prompting another round of the vicious cycle. However, she had never been fully conscious of how all this was linked and this knowledge itself became a catalyst for further change.

If the initial answer you get is framed in the negative (e.g. 'Part of me feels I should be punished'), then ask the following question:

> *What is the positive intention behind X . . . (where X is the negative statement).*

Why is it important to identify the benefits of the problem? Well, if the problems are trying to get something of importance for that person, it is vital that we unearth these and include them in the solution. A smoker may indulge for a variety of positive intentions: to relax (very common), as a time out, to set boundaries, to create a smokescreen, to assert their free will etc. When it comes to preparing for action and then actually taking the steps, we need to have identified other healthy ways by which they can achieve the same benefits. Sometimes this may require learning new skills (relaxation, assertion and so on).

OBSTACLES TO CHANGING

This is the final quadrant to consider. We all put off making changes in different areas of life because of various obstacles that get in the way – both imaginary and real. We may worry about what other people may think or say, mind-reading what their possible negative reactions may be. Drinkers may have real concerns that if they stop drinking and stay clear of the pub, they may lose their friends and other social relationships that alcohol helped them foster. How are they going to fill the gap? This is a major problem in serious drug addictions where stopping the drug may be the easy part. Getting a lifestyle transplant is much harder (new neighbourhood, clean friends, a new job . . .).

You can ask:

> *What obstacles might get in the way of your changing?*

And . . .

> *What's the biggest obstacle that stands in your way?*

Unearthing the biggest obstacle might initially seem to be a counterproductive strategy and decrease motivation for change. However, if this *really is* the biggest obstacle, and you can get round it, reframe it, solve it or resolve it, then nothing else may stand in the way of changing. You can test this by asking:

> *If this really were the biggest obstacle and we solved it, is there anything else that could stand in the way of your taking the first steps?*

You need to look for and welcome this obstacle with open arms and celebrate once you find it. It is often the pivotal point that propels people into preparing for and taking action. We will explore this further in Chapter 10.

Some six months after our initial semi-jocular consultation about smoking, rebellious Rachel had not only sought out more information about smoking cessation, she had decided to 'have a go at stopping'. The way she phrased this statement suggested that certain success was not high on the cards. We explored the obstacles that might get in the way.

She had two major concerns: she used smoking to help her relax and also as a means of social inclusion with her friends. Clearly these were the prime areas where we needed to develop new strategies. She felt that if she could deal with these effectively then her chances of success were much higher.

HELPFUL TASKS

When your patient is in the midst of this stage of ambivalence, the pros and cons of changing can fluctuate throughout their minds and bodies in a way that can feel very frustrating. They can literally feel torn in two. It is often useful to externalise these feelings, to get them out on paper and create a little more emotional distance in order to come to a decision for change to which they are willing to commit. Here are two helpful tasks to ease the way.

Decisional balance sheet

You can create a decisional balance sheet onto which they can write down the answers to all the quadrant questions. It is not simply a matter of stacking up more pros than cons. It is also important to weigh up the emotional intensity attached to each answer and get a feeling for which way the scales are currently tipping. You can give this sheet to your patients to complete at home.

TABLE 8.1 Decisional balance sheet

What would be the greatest benefits of making this change now?	What positive things might this problem actually be doing for me?
What will it cost me in the future if I don't change now?	What obstacles might get in my way?

What's really important to me about making this change?

Ultimately, what would that mean to/for/about me?

Dear diary

For a short period of time, perhaps one or two weeks, keeping a diary of the problem behaviour can provide many useful insights about its occurrence. You are making conscious what was previously on automatic pilot. There is no focus on changing the behaviour, simply noting when it happens, what came immediately before as a potential trigger (events, thoughts, feelings) and what benefits were gained. A diary can be adapted to suit problems such as smoking, binge eating, drinking, drug taking, feelings (anger, anxiety, guilt, etc.), watching television or shopping. Change can often begin to happen through this simple act of observation.

TABLE 8.2 Dear diary

Behaviour monitored:			
Day/Date/Time	Events, thoughts, feelings immediately preceding . . .	Thoughts and feelings during behaviour	Benefits of engaging in the behaviour

Chapter 8 outline summary

Resolving ambivalence
Explore the pros and cons of changing . . . and *not* changing . . . by asking effective questions.

Costs of not changing
- What will it cost you in the future if you don't change now?
- What do you imagine are the worst things that might happen?

Build a vivid, sensory-rich picture of the consequences

Benefits of changing
- What would be the greatest benefits of making this change now?
- Having made the change, what would improve the most?

Build a vivid, sensory-rich picture of the benefits

Benefits of current problem
- What positive things might this problem actually be doing for you?
- What is the positive intention behind the problem behaviour?

Engaging in problem behaviours are often ways of relieving negative feelings that we don't wish to have . . . at least in the short term.

Obstacles that get in the way
- What's the biggest obstacle that stands in your way?
- If this were resolved, would there be anything else that could prevent you from taking the first steps?

Dealing with the biggest obstacle is often the pivotal point in change

Laddering questions
These can be used at any stage to unearth more deeply valued meanings. They connect people to what is really important.
- What's really important to you about that?
- In achieving that, what would that do that is even more important?
- So ultimately, what would this really mean to you?

Helpful tasks
- Decisional balance sheet
- Dear diary

Persuasive phrases

I don't know if you're aware of just how persuasive certain phrases can be when used appropriately. I'm not sure if you've already noticed some of them being used in various chapters thus far. I'd like you to consider that how you choose to use your words can lead people in many different directions. When you fully realise this you will recognise your own skills evolving – exponentially.

During this chapter we are going to explore how particular types of words lend themselves to increasing your influence. This will allow you to begin to use them with volition. In the past you may only have had a surface awareness of the power of certain phrases. By the time you have practised this chapter's contents two or three times you'll find yourself being more persuasive in the future.

Among the many things that people experience in change consultations is an increasing sense of starting to finally head in the direction they really want to go in. When done well it's as if they get an expanding view of what's possible both in terms of ideas and practical action steps. Sometimes the answers seem to arise from within, taking you above and beyond current difficulties. At other times, they're found underneath areas previously overlooked. Persuasive phrases can help the process go more smoothly and effectively.

It may be that you'll naturally start using these phrases by simply having read them. I don't know just how easily you'll recognise doing so. Some people need to practise repeatedly until they finally feel comfortable in their skill level. Usually, however, you'll find that there are one or two phrases that leap out from the page and you can use them immediately to good effect.

You really should take just as much time as you ought to, to become familiar with each category of phrases. You will want to take the time to envisage the kinds of situations in which you intend to utilise them. People often think that they're not supposed to learn things that quickly. Yet you may find that you can readily do just that.

As you read each category you can learn more easily by forming an association in your mind's eye. If you think of a specific situation in the past in which you could have used each phrase then you create a memory peg to hang each one on. Practising in this way causes your learning speed to accelerate dramatically. Doing it in this manner makes subsequent deployment automatic – it becomes second nature.

The fact that you are interested enough to be reading this material means that you are already open to the possibility that you can learn to persuade more effectively. You are beginning to identify with being an active agent of change. Using the strategies you are currently acquiring means that your patients will benefit – sooner than either of you think.

We will take each category in turn, with a brief description and some examples of usage. You can experience what each statement presupposes, what underlying meaning is assumed, and what implications are taken for granted and acted on without thinking. Each of the sentences of all the paragraphs above contains persuasive phrases in action. Once you have learned the categories you can read this section again and spot which phrases belong to each.

AWARENESS

When people have problems their attention is often focused on areas that are less than useful. These words redirect their thoughts to consider things that may not be fully within, or are even entirely beyond, their current awareness. They work well whether you use them with negation or not. Here are examples of some words in this category together with ways to use them.

Aware, notice, consider, think, sense, realise, conceive, perceive . . .

Perhaps you'll consider carefully what I'm about to say . . .

I'm not sure if you've already noticed how much change has occurred so far . . .

Are you aware of just how persuasive these phrases can be . . .

Maybe you've not yet realised that you can persuade with integrity . . .

Now you can make up a few examples of your own.

TIME/TEMPORAL

Experience takes place in the here and now. However, we can use language to access and speak about memories of past experiences and imagine future ones occurring. The implication therefore is that one thing happens after the other in a linear sequence. We can portray this as a line of time extending from the past, through the present and off into the future. Everyone has some way of organising their internal representations of time to make sense of the day-to-day happenings of life. There are many ways that we can use the language of time to manipulate these experiences in a way that promotes change.

The language of time includes verb tenses and numbers:

> Before, during, after, begin, continue, past, present, future, going to, did, had to, will, second, fourth, former, latter . . .

> *You're present here today because you experienced certain things in your past as less than optimal . . .*

> *During our time here today we can begin to explore what you really want . . .*

> *Before you allow yourself to fully experience the change you want to make . . .*

> *The second thing you need to know about changing easily is . . .*

Once again, you can begin to generate your own examples – but only after having decided what you want to presuppose.

SPACE/SPATIAL

Spatial words create relationships and links between things such as thoughts, ideas, people and the services they offer. Change is often a process of separating certain things out and joining other things together. We frequently need to 'ring-fence' or cordon off past hurts, dig up hidden resources and skills and deftly weave them seamlessly into future experiences that become current realities. Space is a powerful metaphor for skilfully sorting out various change issues.

Here are some examples:

> Among, above, below, expanding, beyond, underlying, beside, laying aside, aside from, around, in, on, out of, into . . .

> *Among the many things people experience when changing is a sense of finally moving in the direction they want to go in . . .*

> *Often though, people can literally be beside themselves with the frustration of past failed attempts to change . . .*

Yet sometimes you can find yourself rising above all that and finding that what you really want is just ahead . . .

And I really don't know if the answers will come from inside you or simply arise seemingly unbidden from beyond . . .

ADVERB/ADJECTIVE

Usually, putting adverbs before verbs and adjectives before nouns markedly increases the persuasive impact of the phrases you use. This can help people make changes more easily if they've not yet done so already. Naturally, you'll want to experiment with them yourself to find the best combinations.

Naturally, easily, repeatedly, obviously, finally, accordingly, usually, immediately, readily, truly, already, understandably, some, all . . .

I wonder if you'll find yourself just naturally getting more of what you really want . . .

When you do finally give yourself permission to take the first steps . . .

I don't know how easily you'll notice the changes you're already making . . .

Obviously you'll begin to recognise this when others repeatedly give you positive feedback . . .

POSSIBILITY/NECESSITY

These words imply what we think we can and can't do, what is possible and impossible and what we ought to do instead (or not). In general, whenever we are helping people make changes, we are moving from what may initially be experienced as impossible and opening up to several possible options for doing something different. You can help people get out of very stuck situations and mindframes by skilful use of language. Don't think you ought to do this easily, unless you have already experienced that you can.

Should, have to, must, need, ought, supposed to . . . (and negatives)

Can, will, want, decide, intend, able to . . . (and negatives)

You really should take just as much time as you ought to make this change fit with your circumstances . . .

You know, people often think they're not supposed to change that easily . . .

You can believe on the one hand that change shouldn't be painless . . .

Yet on the other hand you can find you're able to experience it straightforwardly . . .

CAUSE AND EFFECT

We are well used to thinking in terms of one thing causing another to happen. Most of us infer that what we are currently experiencing is a direct result of what has happened in the past. Today's problems are the result of past experiences – so the story goes. Because we are so well versed in automatically thinking this way we can use this structure to create a link between one set of experiences and another – regardless of whether this link was there in the first place or not. If we do this effectively we can generate momentum in the direction of the change we want to make.

The weaker form of linkage: if . . . then, as . . . then, or just 'if' by itself . . .

The stronger form: cause, because, allows, makes, forces, creates, forms, produces, generates, compels, builds, fashions . . .

If you take things one step at a time then change will take place more easily . . .

As you discover your signature strengths then this produces an increasing sense of confidence in your ability to make changes . . .

Thinking about it in this way allows you to create the results you really want . . .

And because you're here today you are already building momentum . . .

MEANING

Meaning is the linguistic glue that holds our realities together and creates identity – *who* we think we are. It implies that one set of experiences and another are synonymous – they mean the same thing. Often people who make mistakes will consider themselves a failure. They confuse a specific behaviour (making a mistake) for an identity statement (I *am* a failure). Because meaning is context-dependent, we can use the skill of reframing to change the associations people make. Changing the meaning in this way prevents people being stuck and frees up the possibility of doing something different instead.

Is, am, are, means, equals, connotes, identify, plus any variation of the verb 'to be' . . .

Your being here today means you're open to changing . . .

Learning new skills means increasing possibilities for change . . .

When you are an agent of change you can persuade people to take action . . .

Helping people get what they really want is a very powerful experience . . .

Remember, you will accelerate your influencing skill by creating your own examples of using persuasive phrases. Even if you spend just a short time refining your expertise your efforts will be repaid handsomely. Your ability to use language effectively is a prime requisite for engaging people in the change process. The more you practise the more successful your results will be.

Interlude 3 outline summary

Certain phrases can be very persuasive when used appropriately. By choosing your words carefully you can lead people in worthwhile directions. Use the categories below to generate many examples.

Awareness

- Aware, notice, consider, think, sense, realise, conceive, perceive . . .

Perhaps you'll carefully consider these words . . . they work with negation or not

Time/temporal

- Before, during, after, begin, continue, past, present, future, going to, did, had to, will, second, fourth, former, latter . . .

Everyone has an internal representation of time to help them make sense of the world

Space/spatial

- Among, above, below, expanding, beyond, underlying, beside, laying aside, aside from, around, in, on, out of, into . . .

Create relationships and links between things such as thoughts, ideas or people

Adverb/adjective

- Naturally, easily, repeatedly, obviously, finally, accordingly, usually, immediately, readily, truly, already, understandably, some, all . . .

Usually, using adverbs and adjectives increases your persuasive impact

Possibility/necessity

- Should, have to, must, need, ought, supposed to . . . (and negatives)
- Can, will, want, decide, intend, able to . . . (and negatives)

You ought to learn how you can put persuasive phrases to work

Cause and effect

- If . . . then, as . . . then, cause, because, allows, makes, forces, creates, forms, produces, generates, compels, builds, fashions . . .

If you use these skills daily then your competency will dramatically increase

Meaning

- Is, am, are, means, equals, connotes, identify, any variation of the verb 'to be' . . .

Increasing competency means increased persuasion power

CHAPTER 9

Preparing to make changes

Whether you and your patients completed the decisional balance sheet on paper or in your mind's eye (*see* Chapter 8), making a decision to proceed with this stage depends largely on the overall benefits of changing outweighing those of staying the same. This preparation phase is absolutely vital to getting the results you want. Skimping here and taking premature, poorly planned action is a recipe for failure. The single most important ingredient for success is a concrete, firm, unyielding state of *commitment*. In fact, from this stage on and throughout the rest of the change process, your patients need an increasing sense of commitment to the task in hand to aid them through the potentially difficult times that can occur – no matter how good the plan.

In preparing, we need to let go of any past focus and begin increasingly to look towards building the kind of future we want to have instead. This phase is solution-centred and must inevitably deal with any obstacles that may crop up. Interestingly, the more specifically we detail the outcome we're after, the more likely we are to unearth the particular obstacles that stand in the way. Metaphorically speaking, it is only when we shine a bright light that the shadows come into sharp relief: the brighter the light, the deeper the shadow. Identifying and dealing with the *right* obstacle is important.

Much of the work of preparation is rehearsal for action. It is mentally imagining and trying on for size different future scenarios and preparing to deal effectively with any obstacles that get in the way. Whether your patients are trying to stop smoking, drinking, overeating, etc., you can bet there will be various environmental triggers (people, places, events, situations), which unleash unresourceful states. Planning in advance how you will deal with a difficult colleague, times of stress, intense cravings etc. can prevent both lapse and relapse.

Whilst it is important to be future oriented, we *can* delve into the past if we do so in a helpful way. We all have various skills and resources that we have picked up along the way. Some of these resources, our *signature strengths*, are the skills, attitudes and mindsets that we have put to good use in other contexts. It is crucial that we unearth these personal strengths and put them to work in the here and now in service of creating the kind of future we want to have.

THE THREE Rs

Preparing to take action is all about building the kind of future we want to have. To do that, we need to get specific about what we want to have happen. We must have a map or operating plan that can guide us, especially when the going gets tough. We need to define our *Results*, the *Reasons* that drive us to achieve them and the *Right action/s* that will get us there.

Results

Too many people fail to define clearly enough the particular result they want in their lives. They tend to speak in generalities, abstractions and about what they don't want rather than specifics of what they do ('I don't want to be depressed, I just want to be happy'). We need to chunk all the way down to the actual behaviours that an observer would see and hear. A key question to ask here is:

> *If someone actually took a video of you getting the result you want, can you describe in detail what's happening . . .?*

Use the following *'what'* questions to further specify the result you want. Remember to get them to step inside the experience as you elicit it.

Box 9.1 Questioning for results

What specific result do you want?
What will let you know you have achieved it?
What will you see, hear and feel as you do that?
What will be different about you then?
When will you do this by (day, date, timeframes etc.)?

When you start to get very precise about the key results you want to have happen in your life it becomes much easier to fill in the details with the particular actions that fit the picture you've painted. You also become clearer about how this fits with other areas of your life and any potential knock-on effects that will have to be dealt with up front. It is much easier to deal with modifications at this stage rather than later.

ROGER'S RESULTS

A key result for Roger, our diabetic, was the ability to go into a restaurant and eat healthy meals commensurate with managing his diabetes well. He pictured himself at business lunches taking a side salad rather than his usual fries with his main order. In place of dessert he opted for a piece of fruit. He saw himself standing up after lunch looking slimmer and telling himself how good it felt to stay on track. Rather than his usual post-lunch energy slump he imagined getting more done as a result. He decided he would start the following Monday.

Reasons

People always do things for a reason. When you think about it, reasons are the motivation, the *why* that provides the impetus for the ensuing action and the perseverance to keep going when setbacks occur. The more 'good reasons' you can bring together to support the result you want, the more motivated you become to take the necessary steps. If you have a big enough *why* then many more things become achievable. For any result you want to create then it is important to become fully aligned with as many powerful reasons as possible. You can get your patients to complete the following statements as a worksheet or simply turn them into face-to-face *why* questions.

Box 9.2 Reasons to get results

I want to get this result because . . .
This result is really important to me because . . .
I am totally committed to getting this result because . . .
I will get this result because . . .
I am capable of getting this result because . . .
I deserve to get this result because . . .
When I get this result I will be able to . . .
Getting this result means that . . .
My purpose in doing this is to . . .
This will benefit others because . . .
Ultimately, succeeding and achieving this result means . . .

It is really useful to write out the answers to these questions in a paragraph. You can keep this with you to remind you of just how important achieving this goal is to you. Whenever you encounter an obstacle your 'why's can connect you with deeply held values that will help you remain firm in your commitment.

ROGER'S REASONS

Roger had several reasons why this result was important to him. He wanted to prove to himself that he still had what it took to make a big decision and stick with it. He was determined to have a different fate to his father's. He reckoned that with his business planning skills he already possessed the capabilities he needed to get started and keep on track. Most of all, with two teenage boys, he wanted to be a positive role model and show them that even after some years of being oblivious to any health concerns he could turn things around.

Right action/s

When you have identified what you want and immersed yourself in the reasons it is important to succeed then the right actions can flow more easily. When you are in this state it becomes much easier to plan what it is you must do to make it happen. Right actions are the 'how to's of successful change. Some actions may be self-evident whilst others may require some brainstorming. You should continue until you have at least half a dozen things you can do. Some of them may be ones you can schedule to do immediately whilst others may need to be done in a certain timeframe.

Smokers may need to set a date, clear the house of any remaining cigarettes and set up a bank account (or piggy bank) to deposit money that would have been otherwise spent on cigarettes. Overeaters may need to clear the fridge of all fattening food, produce a list of healthy groceries to shop for instead and investigate the opening times of the local gym. Drinkers may need to rid the house of alcohol, get in non-alcohol beers instead and avoid going to the pub by setting up other social activities. All may benefit from making a public declaration of their intent. As well as these there may be many other things that are specific to each individual.

Once again you can fill in the following as a worksheet.

Box 9.3 List of right actions I can take

1
2
3
4
5
6
etc . . .

From this list you can get your patient to choose a specific task that they will commit to taking right now. Some of the tasks will need to be broken down into much smaller steps lest they prove overwhelming. A very useful question to ask is:

What is the smallest first step you can commit to taking right now . . .?

Taking small, achievable first steps allows your patients to experience powerful self-reinforcing feelings of success. This will help generate the momentum required when the real action starts in earnest. You can use this question very profitably in the next two stages also.

ROGER'S RIGHT ACTIONS

Roger brainstormed several action steps to help achieve his key result.
> Order side salads and fruit for dessert.
> Ask the chef of his favourite restaurant beforehand to prepare a main course with a 'lighter' sauce.
> One day a week take a packed lunch instead of dining out.
> Take a brisk, 10-minute walk three days a week before lunch.
> Get his kids to ask him how he'd done that day.

GENERATING COMMITMENT

The three Rs are the first steps in generating commitment to take action and make changes that will continue to grow over the rest of the change cycle. If there is no commitment then change will stall. It is therefore highly advantageous to have commitment on tap, especially for the times when problems inevitably crop up. This can make the difference between falling at the first hurdle and crossing the winning line.

We have all experienced the feelings and state of mind and body associated with commitment in the past. When you think about it, you know there have been times when you committed to a particular task and saw it through to a successful conclusion. This has probably occurred in many different contexts in your life: projects at work, various family commitments, perhaps also in sport, hobbies and leisure. In fact, as you look back in time, any goal or task that you have successfully set yourself and completed has involved a promise to yourself to see it through. Your patients will have experienced many similar occasions too.

It is important to be able to reconnect to this state in the here and now and use it in service of maximising the chances of getting the result you want. Here are some questions that will get you in touch with this feeling again. Think about a particular, very specific time in the past when you were really determined to do something and you did it, then answer them.

> **Box 9.4 Generating commitment questions**
>
> When was this occurring . . .?
> Where were you . . .?
> Who else was involved . . .?
> What was happening . . .?
> What does it feel like when you are really committed . . .?
> What do you say to yourself when you're committed in this way . . .?
> How would people know you're committed just by looking at you . . .?
> What would happen if you used this commitment in the current situation . . .?

When people are committed you can see it in their body: the way they hold themselves, their posture, gestures, how they look and what they focus on. You can tell their depth of commitment not only by what they say but also *how* they say it. You can verify this right now by picturing in your mind's eye two people, one of whom is committed, the other laid back and procrastinating. Notice the differences in all these parameters. You can use this as a mental template for gauging the degree of commitment of the person sitting in the consultation chair.

Public commitment

What we have discussed so far is internal commitment – generated by ourselves from the inside. However, making an external commitment can, for some people, pay huge dividends in getting the result they want. There are many ways to do this but here are two that I have found useful.

For smokers in particular I sometimes suggest that they write to five people that they know and respect, telling them of their absolute commitment to be a nonsmoker, naming a date and time when they will accomplish the task. They give an unconditional pledge which, if they fail to live up to, would cause severe loss of face and humiliation. This can be used successfully for many other issues too. It works well for the type of person who has more of an external locus of control and cares about what others think of them. For the self-contained person (internal locus) this is usually a poor motivator.

Many people are motivated by potential loss. You can test this quite easily. If you told someone that by taking a particular action with their bank account they would gain £10 most would not bother to do it, saying it's not worth it for such a small sum. However, if you proceed further and ask them for £10 from their wallet then pretend to rip it up, most will get very upset. The £10 is the same in both cases yet the result is different. That is because whilst we may not be prepared to take action to get something we currently don't have, we are far more engaged when it comes to preventing ourselves from losing out. We can make use of this to persuade someone to take action to get the result they want.

The public commitment in this case is for them to pledge to donate a significant sum of money (or something of equal value in time and energy) if they fail to achieve their goal, to a cause to which they are diametrically opposed. For example, after discussing strategies for weight loss with me, a group of bank employees made various public commitments to help motivate them achieve their target weight. One person who hates cats said he would donate £100 to Cats Protection if he failed. Another, an ardent supporter of Glasgow Celtic football club, committed to buying shares in arch rivals Glasgow Rangers should he fall short. All achieved their targets.

It is really important that the 'donation' be to a group or person that the pledger dislikes (e.g. political party that you loathe). If, for example, you make the donation to a charity you like then you will still feel good if you fail to get your result because a 'good cause' will have benefited instead. This may reduce your efforts in changing your behaviour. It is a far more powerful motivator to think you are losing something you really value to a cause you despise. Try it and see.

DEALING WITH OBSTACLES

The more you refine the details of the result you want to make happen the more likely it is that obstacles will show up on the path. Many clinicians get a sinking feeling when obstacles turn up. They believe that they may derail the whole change process. Sometimes they try to either avoid or minimise them. This is not a useful strategy.

It is really important to actively seek out potential obstacles in advance. If they are likely to stop your patient in their tracks in the real world outside your consulting room, then it's best that you prepare them to deal with them beforehand. In fact you should rejoice when you hit obstacles. They are the very things that help you fine-tune the result your patient wants and actually increase the likelihood of long-term success. In truth, when you find the biggest obstacle, the prime objection that stands in the way, then you are only one reframe away from helping them get the change they want and deserve.

What people want is not necessarily what they expect will happen. I have found it very useful to incorporate the following question to flush out the objections that are likely to rise along the path:

> Given that this is the result you want . . . what do you expect is actually going to happen?

Usually they will begin to tell you their success story, which shortly runs into a brick wall. For a smoker it could be plain sailing until the 'work's night out' when they have had a drink or two and are susceptible to offers of a cigarette. For the binge drinker it may be when a certain 'mate' comes calling with a six-pack. For the shopaholic it may be when they pass a certain store. For the diabetic it may be a particular aisle of 'goodies' in the supermarket. For the overweight person who really wants to exercise it may be coming home tired after a busy day at work when the television and couch – and bag of crisps – speak more seductively than the gym.

You can also ask:

> *What are the main obstacles you think will get in the way of achieving your result?*

And, of course, the follow-up question to both is:

> *What strengths, skills, attitudes, behaviours, etc. will you really need to overcome these obstacles?*

The key element, then, is to discover the particular roadblock they are likely to run into and determine just what specific tactic they need to deal with it successfully. Then you can help them find just which one of their signature strengths will pay dividends just when they need it.

IDENTIFYING AND UTILISING SIGNATURE STRENGTHS

We have all had times in the past when we created something, we achieved a particular result that was important to us, and turned what was a dream into reality. Perhaps you went after a particular job and got it. Maybe you decided to move house and did. You possibly even planned and organised a major holiday to a place you'd always wanted to go. Perhaps you saved enough money to buy that special present for a loved one. Maybe there was a particular time when you thought you were going to fail yet you surprised yourself by rising to the occasion and succeeding. Often we take these things for granted. It is as if we have forgotten our past successes or just gloss over them deprecatingly. Yet within those past successes lies the very core of our signature strengths.

Get your patients (and yourself) to list several achievements that stand out for them over the years. Go through every decade of their life so far and find at least two things from each time period that were personal triumphs, successes or accomplishments. Include all contexts of life – work, family, relationships, finance, sports, hobbies etc. Focus especially on late teenage years and into the twenties. This is when people often had a lot of vision and energy to actually get something done. You may have to assist some patients to reframe their ideas of what success looks like to help them notice their achievements. You can do this conversationally during a consultation. Or you can, as a homework exercise, make sure they fill out the sheet below.

Box 9.5 My list of personal achievements in my life

1

2

3

4

5

6

7

8

9

10

For each of the achievements you unearth, dust off and breathe life into again, you can ask:

Box 9.6 Achievement questions

What did you do to achieve this?

How did you actually make it happen?

What steps did you take?

What did you focus on?

How did you deal with any obstacles that got in the way?

Then from the list below, select which personal strengths they used to achieve these tasks. The very act of recording the successes, questioning how they made them come about and perusing the list itself will start to regenerate the feelings associated with those times.

CHART 9.1 Signature strengths

adaptable	alive	ambitious	assertive	assured
bold	brave	calm	capable	caring
challenging	committed	compassionate	courageous	creative
curious	decisive	dependable	determined	dignified
diligent	dynamic	eager	effective	energetic
enthusiastic	excited	fascinated	fearless	flexible
focused	forgiving	forward looking	friendly	full of fun
glamorous	graceful	grateful	happy	healthy
helpful	honest	hopeful	imaginative	ingenious
innovative	inspired	intelligent	jovial	joyful
keen	kind	knowledgable	learning easily	loving
loyal	luscious	masterful	mature	optimistic
ordered	organised	passionate	peaceful	persevering
playful	powerful	problem solving	relaxed	reliable
resilient	resourceful	revolutionary	safe	secure
sharing	solid	stimulated	strong	successful
trustworthy	truthful	unique	unstoppable	useful
vital	wise	witty	worthy	zealous

Once again, it can be very useful to give your patients a photocopied list of all these strengths, which they can take home with them and scrutinize at their leisure. In the consultation itself, though, you may want to get one or two words which typify them at their best. Having identified them you can ask the signature strength questions.

> **Box 9.7 Signature strength questions**
>
> What does it feel like when you are really X . . .? (Where X is the strength)
> What do you focus on in your mind's eye when you're X?
> What do you say to yourself when you're X in this way . . .?
> What kind of posture and gestures do you have when you are X?
> How would people know you're X . . . just by looking at you . . .?
> What would happen if you used this X when you meet an obstacle . . .?

Putting strengths to work

Once you have found and reclaimed this person's individual strengths, it's time to put them to work. You can get them to conjure up in their imagination the likely obstacles that could derail them and watch how differently things turn out when they apply what they have just learned in this situation. Have them imagine it both from outside in and inside out. That is, get them to step into the experience as if it's happening now and ensure it goes the way they want it to. If it doesn't then that is simply a cue to remind you to dust off another signature strength and try it on for size instead.

Utilising signature strengths is probably the quickest way to give someone a sense of an inner locus of control in a situation. It lets them know that they now have a genuine response-ability. They may not have all the answers but they now have a self-reinforcing mechanism that they can use in many different situations.

It is really useful to give patients a homework exercise to identify as many strengths as possible and run them through the questioning process. When you give people the chance to reconnect to themselves in this way, the positive effects can extend way into the future, well beyond your present encounter. Of course, you can continue to use this exercise in the final two stages of change when appropriate.

DEALING WITH ROGER'S OBSTACLES

Roger could see everything going to plan in the restaurant until it came to desserts. With his sweet tooth he knew he would find it difficult to resist, especially if his business colleague was having one. This could be his Achilles heel.

Many years earlier he had been a rugby wing forward playing at district level. He had scored many tries but the one that gave him most pleasure was at the interdistrict championships when his underrated team had run out narrow winners. He cited his drive, focus and ability to keep going against the odds as key strengths.

When Roger relived that specific memory and answered the signature strength questions, he was surprised how easily the positive feelings surfaced and how good it made him feel. The word 'Drive!' seemed to galvanise him with energy. He imagined shouting it out inside his mind (not out loud!) when the dessert menu arrived and thought that this would definitely help him to more easily resist.

Chapter 9 outline summary

The three Rs

- *Results* – What you want and how you will know you've achieved it
- *Reasons* – The 'Why' that provides the impetus for action
- *Right action/s* – The specific steps you are committed to taking

What is the smallest first step you can commit to taking right now?

Generating commitment

Commitment is one of the most important states in both this and the subsequent stages. An increasing sense of commitment maximises chances of success.

- Ask the 'generating commitment' questions
- Attach the state to each of the right actions
- Get people to make public commitments, especially if they have an external locus of control

Dealing with obstacles

Seek out potential obstacles in advance so you can deal with them effectively

- What are the main obstacles you think will get in the way of achieving your result?
- What strengths, skills, attitudes, behaviours, etc. will you need to overcome this?

Signature strengths

The skills, behaviours, beliefs and values that are true of you when you are at your best

- List your top 10 achievements so far
- Ask 'achievement' questions to find out how you made this happen
- Ask 'signature strength' questions to reconnect to these powerful resources
- Put the strengths to work by connecting them to the three Rs

Emotional messages

Emotions are systemic states that encompass our thinking and feeling as well as have direct effects on our physiology and behaviours. It is impossible to go through a process of change without encountering potentially strong emotions along the way. Although emotions can be both positive (joy, gratitude, pleasure etc.) and negative (fear, anger, sadness etc.), it is usually the negative ones that seem to create most problems. People vary in their capacity to cope with emotions and attempt to deal with them in different ways.

Some people try to avoid negative emotions altogether by exiling them from their awareness. They do not want to accept the pain that invariably accompanies them and thus avoid risk taking in the hope of remaining safe and secure. Inevitably, though, this excess caution generates more suffering rather than less. Given that it is impossible not to experience emotions such as fear and sadness, by remaining stoical we run the risk of pushing them underground, even repressing them. Studies show quite clearly that harbouring negative feelings such as depression over the long term can lead to immune system dysfunction and heart disease.

Other people may feel their feelings very intensely and passionately express them at every opportunity. Sometimes this is done with volition, at others like an exploding bomb. Occasionally it may seem as if they are engaging in a competition – *let me tell you just how bad I feel*. It is a strange paradox that some people may have a sense of pride that they feel worse than someone else – and beware anyone who tries to help them out of it. Rather than doing something about their negative emotions they may be content to endure or even wallow in them.

Every emotion that we have, both positive and negative, is useful and can serve us in some way. To be emotionally intelligent we need to recognise and manage them both in ourselves and in our relationships with others. We need to develop our capacity for unearthing the meaning and message each emotion portrays and utilise it as a way of motivating ourselves to take action and make changes. Given that emotions are impossible to avoid, we must adopt a different strategy to stoicism or explosion. Treating them as important non-verbal signals is a key step in the change process.

We will examine the common negative emotions in turn and find out how we can intelligently express their underlying implications. When we do this effectively we will find that so-called negative emotions have a positive message which, when expressed, will let the overwhelming feelings rapidly subside as we take productive action.

FEAR

Fear, and its lesser derivatives anxiety and worry, occur when we think that something bad will happen in the future. We foresee negative consequences that we want to avoid. We may think we are going to lose something we value or fail to achieve our desired result. Unfortunately, as these images loom large in our thinking, the accompanying feelings can prevent us from taking effective action. We can feel out of control, victimised by circumstances and rather impotent in the face of impending disaster.

Many people fear making changes. To do so requires movement from a place of seeming safety, security and comfort into a world where anything might go wrong. The fear may be due to the potential risk of physical and emotional consequences – pain and humiliation or embarrassment. It can also arise from challenges to deeply held beliefs and values that may call in to question our sense of self or identity. Sometimes the fear is due to a major concern that we may be at risk of actual physical harm. If that is really the case, then we need to take avoiding action promptly. Mostly, though, it is because we have blown things out of proportion.

The underlying message of fear is that there is something coming up for which we have to prepare effectively. It is important not to ignore any negative consequences. However, rather than blowing things out of proportion we need to step back, gain perspective on the situation and decide what effective actions we can take instead to get what we want. We must develop an effective plan that covers all the bases.

Even when we have decided what needs to be done we may still feel uncomfortable and reticent. This is when we need to take our courage in both hands and commit to moving forwards. Often the simple act of taking the first step dispels the residual tensions. We can then be open to the ever-present, ongoing feedback that helps us refine our actions.

The most important questions to answer then are:

What specifically are you fearful of . . .?

How can you reduce the negative consequences . . .?

What do you need to do instead . . .?

ANGER

Anger occurs when an important rule or boundary has been violated. Perhaps someone has behaved inappropriately and put at risk something we value. This can be at a physical or emotional level and also be about our beliefs and identity. When people hold different views of the world from ours, there is great potential for conflict if we insist that our views are the only correct and allowable interpretation. The more rules we have, and the more rigid these are, the more likely we will experience anger on an ongoing basis.

Although anger is an intense and often brief emotion, if unresolved it can lead to feelings of frustration, resentment and hatred. This can then lead to a sense of vulnerability, insecurity and victimhood which perpetuates a negative cycle. We may explode at others inappropriately or, in an effort to avoid anger altogether, distance ourselves from the things that are important to us to avoid getting hurt. Neither approach yields dividends.

The message of anger, then, is to allow us to re-establish our boundaries and rules. Before we can do that, we need to be clear that not only has a violation taken place but that our rules are actually worth sticking up for. Sometimes we are responding out of the distant past when our rules were based on authority figures of our younger years. We therefore have an opportunity to check that these rules remain appropriate and, if not, to establish new rules. If they do remain appropriate then we need to uphold them respectfully.

When we effectively express our anger in this way we preserve our personal integrity and maintain our boundaries. By mounting a legitimate complaint we give other people the chance to repair any damage and prevent any reoccurrence. Even if they don't, we can maintain the satisfaction of doing whatever we are capable of to sustain our values.

Effective questions are:

What specifically are you angry about . . .?

What rule has been broken . . .?

Is this worth upholding . . .?

What do you need to do to re-establish your boundaries . . .?

GUILT

In a sense, guilt is anger directed against oneself. When we do something that we feel we shouldn't have, causing either ourselves or someone else to suffer, then we violate our own rules and disrupt any equanimity we may have had. Guilt is based on the judgment that we have gone against what is deeply important to us and caused unwanted and unlooked for consequences.

Guilt is an emotion that motivates us to address a problem. Yet if we fail to do so we may become pessimistic, remorseful and may even end up in deep self-loathing and depression. We may become fearful that our 'mistake' will be discovered, become even more insecure and much less likely to admit our errors. Oftentimes we mistakenly identify with the problem behaviour – instead of resolving the situation *we* become 'bad' rather than the errant behaviour itself.

The message of guilt, then, is that we have transgressed and must make amends for our behaviour. Perhaps this requires an apology, maybe a specific action of atonement or recommitment. This can be either to another person or even to ourselves. By doing so, we restore our dignity and integrity and realign with our values. If we have violated another person in some way then we have the opportunity to repair the mistake and re-establish the relationship.

Questions to ask are:

What specifically do you feel guilty about . . .?

Which of your rules or values have you violated . . .?

What do you need to do to make amends . . .?

What is the first step you can take right now . . .?

SADNESS

Sadness and grief usually occur when we have lost something that we value highly. This can be loss of a person as in bereavement and also such things as loss of a job, prized possession, even a dream we once had. Whilst sadness is often an emotion about a past loss we can also feel sad about an impending loss in the future.

If we try to avoid or deny sadness, pretending it doesn't exist or distancing ourselves from it, we may become shut down and experience even less of all the other emotions available to us. Life can become cold and empty. When we cling to a past that can never return and continue to mourn our loss we remain deeply enmeshed with the lost object. We cut ourselves off more and more from the outside world and shut off to any future possibilities.

Sadness can be a key emotion at any time of personal change. When we transition from one part of our life to the next we invariably leave something behind. If people have had intimate relationships with food, alcohol, cigarettes or drugs, then the void left behind by their absence can be very hard to fill. It is the pulling power of the vortex of this void that causes so many to lapse and relapse.

In preparing to make any change we must endeavour to bring every healthy positive association that belonged to the lost object into the future. Given that it is the feelings generated by this object that we grieve, we must reclaim these feelings from it and incorporate them into daily life. Sometimes this will require a period of mourning and perhaps a ritual to lay the object finally to rest. In all change processes it is important to identify and preserve the underlying positive aspects and benefits of the problem situation and integrate them into any proposed solution.

Useful questions to ask are:

Who or what specifically are you sad about . . .?

What is it that you feel you have lost . . .?

How can you bring these positive associations with you into the future . . .?

What ritual will help you to honour the past and move on . . .?

SHAME

Shame is a very close relative of guilt and they often go hand in hand. We all tend to project a particular image that we want other people to see as us. Shame occurs when we have an inner fear that we don't match up to this outer image and, worse still, our shortcomings may be made public and expose us to ridicule or embarrassment. We feel we are not as good as we try to be. Secret drinkers may use alcohol to help them portray apparent confidence and bonhomie, yet underneath it all be struggling with inner demons.

All shame is based on false self-identification. It leads to self-devaluation, self-degradation and perhaps deep depression. This global lack of self-esteem insidiously permeates all facets of life and becomes the root of all negative evaluations. Everything is magnified, often out of all proportion. Trivial errors become overwhelming judgments and indictments of grave shortcomings.

The underlying message of shame is to make us aware that our inner and outer realities are at odds with each other. Recognising that allows us to do something effective about it. If it arises from guilt then we may need to apologise and make amends both to self and others. If shame is due to self-devaluation and inferiority it draws attention to the fact that our self-image is in need of revision. The call is for increasing self-acceptance, and an ability to detach and let go of false images. This is often hard to do for oneself and may require professional help. However the palpable relief we experience when we stop pretending to be something we're not and drop the façade is immeasurable.

We can also uncover the underlying positive intention that this façade is trying to achieve for us. This intention is often a feeling of confidence and inner strength. These are personal resources and states of mind and body that can be unearthed, revivified and put to work. You will find more on the vital aspects of discovering and working to build signature strengths in Chapter 10.

Questions to ask include:

What specifically do you feel ashamed of . . .?

Which rules or values have you violated . . .?

How can you make amends . . . to others . . . to yourself . . .?

What does this façade do for you that's important . . .?

How can you develop this resource more effectively instead . . .?

What we have dealt with so far are five of the major negative emotions that can get in the way of persuading someone to make personal changes. We will go on to deal with some of the lower-intensity but just as pervasive feelings that can occur on a daily basis when you are engaged in going for a result you want to make happen.

FRUSTRATION

Frustration occurs when you believe you should be better at something than you currently are. You have set a particular goal but for some reason you are not making the headway you think you ought to. Sometimes there are external obstacles that prevent us getting what we want. Sometimes the obstacle is ourselves – our recurrent patterns of thinking, feeling and behaving.

It is hard to feel frustrated if you don't know where you're heading. This is an emotion that can only occur when you are on route to a change that hasn't yet happened. It can only occur if you've already engaged in moving towards a key result you've decided to act on. In this way frustration is an important signal letting you know that what you're doing isn't working. You may have to take on board new information, change direction, or do something different.

Key questions are:

What specific obstacles are getting in your way . . .?

What information are you currently lacking . . .?

What do you need to do differently to get the result you want . . .?

What is the first step you can take right now . . .?

DISAPPOINTMENT

Disappointment is another emotion that can only occur if you have begun to engage in the change process. It signals that you have missed out on achieving the result you wanted to make happen. Put simply, if you didn't make any plans then you wouldn't feel disappointed. As soon as you have expectations of success then disappointment is always lurking on the sidelines to help you fine-tune your plans.

You can be let down when other people don't fulfil their agreed part in helping you get your outcome. You can also let yourself down – by having expectations that are unrealistic or finding that you lack the necessary skills. This is a key message about ensuring that you are not totally dependent on others to achieve your goals and that you yourself have the right skills in hand to tackle the situation. It is important that you see disappointment for what it is – an opportunity to review what has happened, learn any lessons, refine your goals and reformulate a new action plan.

Some questions to ask:

What specifically are you disappointed about?

What lessons can you learn from this . . .?

What refinements will you make to your original goal . . .?

What skills will you use to achieve this result . . .?

OVERWHELM

Many people want to make changes, fail to plan adequately, jump straight in at the deep end and find themselves rapidly overwhelmed if not drowning. Others don't even take the first step. They experience themselves as victims at the mercy of a powerful external world. Their problems loom large and appear insoluble – so much so that it looks like there's nothing they can do.

Feelings of overload and overwhelm can quickly turn into more prolonged stress and even depression. When there is too much to handle we may give up, disengage and let the storm break around us. If we are not careful we may not even do the small, simple things that help us take care of ourselves. In the midst of so much to deal with we end up doing nothing at all.

Overwhelm is a signal that there are too many things happening at once – we need to prioritise. It is a message that we need to re-establish an internal locus of control by paying attention to the most important thing that we can do right now. Of all the things that are happening right now, which one is key? It is often useful to write down a list of everything you are dealing with. Getting this down on paper externalises it, reduces the negative feelings and starts to bring back a sense of control. Of course it is vital to differentiate between what is really in your control and what is merely wishful thinking.

Here are some useful questions.

What are all the things that are overwhelming you . . .?

Out of all of these, which ones are within your control . . .?

And from these, which is the most important one to focus on now . . .?

What is the first step you can take . . .?

Emotions play a large part in the change process. They can arise unexpectedly in any of the stages of change. And without some degree of emotional input, change may well be very difficult. The negative emotions we have discussed above often tend to get in the way – they produce a lot of steam at times for little forward action. However when you unearth the oft-times simple message underlying them, the reframed content releases the energy for useful work – metaphorically speaking. When people can view what once was a marked emotional reaction both with a sense of equanimity and as a spur for moving in a new direction, then you will have done your job well.

Although I have not explicitly discussed positive emotions here, you can use the same process to establish deeply meaningful connections to underlying messages.

Interlude 4 outline summary

Emotional messages
- Emotions are systemic states that encompass our thinking and feeling as well as having direct effects on our physiology and behaviours
- Emotional intelligence means recognising and effectively utilising the underlying message of any emotions that arise

Fear

- Foreseeing negative consequences that we want to avoid
- We need to prepare effectively with the information available
- *Ask – What do you need to do instead?*

Anger

- Occurs when an important rule or boundary has been violated
- Check if the rule is still worth upholding or needs updating
- *Ask – What do you need to do to respectfully reassert your boundaries?*

Guilt

- Occurs when we violate our own rules and boundaries
- We may feel we deserve punishment for our actions
- *Ask – What amends do you need to make?*

Sadness

- We have lost something that is highly valued
- It is a key emotion in times of personal change
- *Ask – What ritual will help you honour the past and move on?*

Shame

- Fear that our shortcomings may be made public and we are 'exposed'
- Often results from a negative self-image and self-devaluation
- *Ask – How can you safely drop this façade and become more resourceful?*

Frustration

- Occurs when obstacles (internal and external) prevent goal achievement
- What you are doing isn't working and needs changing
- *Ask – What do you need to do differently to get the result you want?*

Disappointment

- You have missed out on achieving the result you wanted to make happen
- Your expectations must be realistic and not entirely dependent on others
- *Ask –What refinements will you make to your original goal?*

Overwhelm

- There are too many things happening at once and you feel out of control
- You must re-establish an internal locus of control by prioritising
- *Ask – What is the most important thing to focus on right now?*

CHAPTER 10

Taking action

This is the stage that most of us equate with *really* changing. It is when, to the external world at least, most of the activity (often frenetic), seems to take place. It is a busy stage and may require much support. Yet because it is such a seductive stage – we are released into doing many things at once which can be gratifying – if it is not founded upon adequate preparation beforehand, it is doomed to failure.

Premature action often ensues 'the morning after the night before'. Too many drinks or cigarettes, too much food, a huge credit card bill, engaging in risky behaviour, etc., may leave such a feeling of distaste that no sooner have the immortal words 'never again' left our lips then we are rashly planning to make major changes tomorrow – or earlier. Such action generally fizzles out within a few days to a week and may repeat itself cyclically every few weeks to months. This leads to a very frustrating and depressing yo-yo effect, especially if you are a crash dieter.

Others may want you, the clinician, to wave a magic wand and have the change miraculously happen without any effort on their part. I do keep a magic wand in my drawer yet its exhibition rarely has the desired effect – other than laughter. Some may want you to hypnotise them so that when they awaken the problem will be gone. Change requires action and effort, which may need to be sustained over many weeks and even months. Some people are simply just not ready – others don't want to invest the time and energy.

Your patients may be taking action for the *n*th time. Yet they may be using exactly the same methodologies, strategies, techniques and approaches that ultimately failed the last time – and the time before that. It's as if only they could try harder or for longer then surely it will work out this time. What they fail to do is to learn from past failures. They may need exposure to new approaches and techniques, perhaps even several different ones sequentially or simultaneously, to get the result they want. There are many to choose from and not one of them has a monopoly on successful change.

Taking action is all about marshalling your resources and energies and keeping them pointed for long enough in the right direction until the change you want to make becomes bedded in – and as automatic as the problem used to be. It is about using the commitment already generated in the preparation phase as a platform to launch and sustain your action plan. It is about repeatedly bringing your signature strengths into play to drive change forwards.

Since what we often call problem behaviour is, more often than not, the result of trying to get away from negative feelings and emotions and move towards pleasure – no matter how short-lived (drugs, alcohol, food, cigarettes) – it is very useful to look at this stage through the lens of recurring states of mind and body. We need to actively manage our states on a day-to-day basis to ensure we are in the right state for the job in hand. Much of this chapter will be about how to ensure your patients – and you yourself – can remain focused and energised during this challenging period.

STATES AND ENERGY

All feelings, emotions and states of mind and body are intimately connected to energy. States, whether positive or negative, have both an energy level and a direction of flow associated with them. For example, revulsion has energy that pushes us away from something whilst attraction has a completely different feel as it pulls us towards something else. It is possible to sort states out into four basic categories depending on their degree of positivity versus negativity and high versus low energy.

Low energy, negative states

States such as boredom, depression, hopelessness and helplessness are all negative states with a low energy. They feel very uncomfortable to be in and are often difficult to get out of easily. They keep people stuck – like wading through treacle. They are major obstacles to taking action of any kind and are to be avoided in this stage of changing. The classic way out is through the previously conditioned and engrained problem behaviour (just have a cigarette or a drink or two and forget about it all). This is a revolving door predicament leading to a lapse or relapse. We need to ensure that our patients either avoid going there or have some way out. We will shortly look at ways of interrupting this pattern and getting into and maintaining higher energy positive states.

High energy, negative states

Anger, fear, anxiety and panic are the classic high-energy negative states. Slightly less energetic but still debilitating are states such as frustration and exasperation. Rather than heeding the message buried within the emotion (*see* Interlude 4), we try to tranquillise it away with our 'drug of choice'. We want to get into lower

High Energy, Negative State	High Energy, Positive State
Anger	In the Flow
Fear	Confident
Anxiety	Enthusiastic
Panic	Invigorated
Frustration	Powerful
Exasperation	Dynamic
Dissatisfaction	Resourceful
Low Energy, Negative State	Low Energy, Positive State
Boredom	Relaxed
Depression	Calm
Overwhelm	Peaceful
Hopelessness	Meditative
Helplessness	Mellow
Defeated	Serene
Dejected	Equanimity

FIGURE 10.1 States and energy

energy, positive states and this is often what problem behaviour attempts to do for us – at a price. We need to develop more legitimate means of accessing these relaxing states, of 'chilling out', which is often difficult to do directly. Oddly enough, it is often easier to make a detour via the higher-energy positive states first.

Low energy, positive states

These are comfortable, peaceful, relaxed states, which many people are searching for, yet may not have direct access to without artificial assistance. They are regenerative states of mind and body. Thoughts slow down and may simply murmur in the background. Bodily processes slow down too – heart rate and breathing decelerate to an easy rhythm. The parasympathetic nervous system takes over, stress levels reduce and healing takes place. We need to help people establish simple rituals that allow them to reach this place easily.

High energy, positive states

These are great states to live out of on a daily basis. It is difficult to engage in problem behaviour when we are already feeling confident, enthusiastic and resourceful. The higher levels of energy and positive outlook allow us to get more done, effectively, and feel good about ourselves (remember Barbara Fredrickson, page 18). It also helps us connect and interact more successfully with others – even if we previously didn't. Much of the time, many problem behaviours are trying to get us into this quadrant, yet fall short of the mark. It is important to develop mini-rituals and practices that allow us to generate these states at will more frequently.

CHANGING STATES

From the foregoing it is clear that a major and universal requirement for anyone involved in making changes, no matter what the underlying issues and problems, is the ability to move quickly from negative to positive states. Developing and maintaining positive states is a key plank in building a stable platform to successfully launch the other strategies in this chapter. Firstly, we need to have a robust way of getting out of high- and low-energy negative states before moving to resourcefulness or relaxation.

Pattern interrupts

We can envisage both low- and high-energy negative states as a series of thinking and behavioural patterns, which lead inexorably to feeling stuck. Whilst there are many ways to change stuck states we want to spend as little time as possible both in the state itself, and in the getting out of jail process. We need a ritual that will effect the change in as little as a few seconds and at the most a few minutes. We need something that will interrupt the negative pattern and stop it in its tracks.

One of the quickest ways to change state is to change our physiology – our postures, gestures and movements. Each state of mind and body comes pre-packaged as it were, with a particular body posture, set of movements, energetic rhythm and voice tone. You can easily check this out. Imagine in your mind's eye someone who is depressed and lethargic. Notice how they are moving, where their gaze is focused and how their voice sounds. Now imagine someone who is confident and dynamic. How are they different?

We can put this difference to work immediately.

Box 10.1 Pattern interrupts

Imagine that you feel strong, dynamic, powerful, unstoppable, with every skill you have instantly accessible.

Act as if this is happening right now.

Pretend that you can easily do this.

Imagine what your body position and posture is like in this state.

Put yourself in exactly the same body position and posture.

Repeatedly use a gesture that typifies this state.

Say over and over in your inner ear the words that epitomise it.

Adopt an attitude and feeling of complete and utter certainty.

Move around whilst you allow the feelings to grow even stronger.

One of my favourite ways to immediately get out of an unresourceful state is to adopt a karate posture and do a few high-energy moves. Within 10 seconds my state has changed markedly for the better. I suggest you think of ways in which you can change your state quickly – and get your patients to do so too. Other ways can include: dancing to your favourite music or song, shadow boxing, callisthenics, having a shower, phoning a friend, jogging on the spot, skipping and jumping, walking the dog, etc. etc. Get your patients to fill in various ways to instantly change state from this section and the next and write them down.

Box 10.2 Ways to instantly change state

1

2

3

4

5

6

7

8

9

10

We need to give a special mention to aerobic exercise. This has been shown in many studies to reduce both anxiety and depression and enhance body image and self-esteem. It causes the direct release of endorphins, the brain chemicals that reduce pain and increase our sense of well-being. There are many ways to reach your aerobic threshold for 20–30 minutes or so, three or four times a week – daily is even better. They include swimming, cycling, jogging, dancing, plus the various cardiovascular machines found in gyms. I often suggest to depressed patients that they burn a 20-minute CD of their favourite upbeat music and dance to it each day.

Changing focus

As well as making physical changes, we can change our state by changing our mental focus. When we are in negative states our internal thoughts and imagery often keep us stuck in a vicious cycle of conflict and discomfort. We picture how badly things are going, tell ourselves it's getting worse, and feel even more awful. It is not very easy to go directly from negative to positive imagery in one step. We need to have a method of disengagement which gets us out of the negativity first before re-engaging with positive thoughts. We can do this first by using a *distancing* process.

Box 10.3 Distancing from negative thought processes

Make an image in your mind's eye of your current negative experience.
Step out of the image and picture 'that you' over there (dissociate).
Make the image like a still-frame photograph.
Imagine making it shrink down and move further away beyond arm's reach.
Make the image black and white, dull or even fuzzy and out of focus.
Turn down the volume of any sounds, making them quieter and more distant.

If you repeat this process several times with your negative imagery, moving the picture further away each time, then you will find the associated negative feelings diminishing. Even if you are one of those people who can't see internal images very well, the process will work equally well if you simply pretend or make believe that each step is happening. Some people like to use a physical gesture as if they're grabbing hold of the picture and firmly pushing it away from them. This gives them the feeling of being more in control.

Now we can re-engage with higher-energy, more positive feelings associated with resourceful imagery. You can start by imagining what you would look like if you were dynamic, powerful, invigorated and confident. Notice how you would walk, talk, breathe and move feeling this way. You can intensify this positive imagery by doing the following steps.

Box 10.4 Enhancing positive emotions

Make an image in your mind's eye of this positive experience – dynamic, powerful, invigorated, confident.
Step fully into 'that you' as if it's happening now.
Make the image into a movie.
Imagine everything getting bigger, brighter and coming closer.
Intensify the colours and see everything clearly and brightly.
Turn up the volume of any sounds and imagine it as 'surround sound'.

It is well worth your effort practising this several times before you need to use it. Doing so will dramatically enhance the positive associations. You can also use your own real-life past memories that you greatly value to boost you further – perhaps times when you achieved something of importance, memories of great holidays, happy occasions such as the birth of a child, etc. In fact, any memory that you personally value very highly will benefit from this kind of 'facelift'. You can also give your memories a one- or two-word label so that, in time, just saying the word will bring back the good feelings – exactly when you need them.

Relaxing rituals

Learning how to relax just when you need to is a skill well worth mastering. Many of the habits we want to give up are actually trying to attain relaxation for us. The classic of course is when someone feels frazzled and is desperate for a cigarette. A couple of really long 'drags' and relaxation descends. This gives us a major clue. The deep diaphragmatic breaths invoke the relaxation response by triggering the parasympathetic nervous system. The trick, of course, is to invoke the response without the cigarette.

Breathing is one of the bodily processes which, although it occurs automatically and usually out of awareness, can also be controlled consciously. Most negative states (and positive ones too) have typical breathing patterns associated with them. Anxiety, anger and agitation usually involve breathing high in the chest with short breaths, the in-breath being the same length or even longer than the out-breath. Relaxation is the complete opposite. Breaths are much slower, arise from the abdomen, and the out-breath is much longer in duration than the in-breath. We can use our conscious mind override to deliberately invoke the relaxation response whenever we need it. Find a quiet place where you can be undisturbed for 10 minutes and do the following process.

Box 10.5 Relaxation response

Settle yourself comfortably making sure your clothes are loose.
Close your eyes.
Become aware of your feet, your calf muscles and your thighs.
Focus on each out-breath from now on.
Lengthen the out-breath so it lasts much longer than the in-breath.
Notice if you can let it last twice as long.
Notice your abdomen moving out and in.
Do this for 10–20 breaths.
Then start from the beginning again to deepen your relaxation.

Once you have done this a few times then it becomes automatic. You will find that even in the midst of a potentially stressful and overwhelming period at work or home, simply taking a moment or two to take a couple of relaxing breaths will reduce your arousal levels considerably. Of course it is always a good idea to practise beforehand in settings that are potential triggers for negative states so that you more easily maintain an inner locus of control. For those people interested in developing relaxation skills further, then classes in yoga, tai chi, meditation, hypnosis etc., may be beneficial.

In summary then, pattern interrupts, distancing from the negative, enhancing the positive and learning the relaxation response are four fundamental skills for anyone involved in taking action. You can use them in the order given so that you can more easily move from negative to positive states in the most effective way possible. You can begin to plan to live each day more in the high-energy positive states with short forays into relaxation to ensure balance.

You will be aware that I have written this section as if addressed specifically to you the reader. As the agent of change it is important that you master all the above techniques and use them when appropriate. Remember to teach them to your patients too.

RACHEL'S SMOKING HABIT

Rachel made great use of the techniques in this section to help her with her major obstacles in overcoming her smoking habit. Her principal obstacle had been using a cigarette to help her relax when she was frequently harassed. She had found it easier than she had originally thought to cut out many of the cigarettes that she habitually and almost mindlessly lit up just through simple awareness. However, half a dozen or so remained deeply entrenched. They were the ones that quickly allowed her to unwind and calm down when feeling stressed.

She developed the following ritual, which she initially perfected at home before finding herself automatically using it at work. Whenever she found herself 'feeling frazzled' she closed her eyes and imagined putting all of the negativity into a black bin-liner, which she sealed tightly. Then she envisaged swinging it round and round her head before launching it off into space to diminish into a small dot in the distance. She did the same with any residual feelings until they had diminished to manageable proportions. Then she focused on the relaxation response by exhaling 10 slow breaths whilst she concentrated on her feet, calves and thighs.

She finished off by visualising a stream of positive energy entering the soles of her feet and going up to the top of her head. She gave this an orange colour and imagined it filling her up completely. She accompanied this with the soundtrack of her favourite upbeat pop song so that by the time she opened her eyes she was ready to get going again. This short ritual streamlined quickly with practice so that it took less than 30 seconds to complete.

Although she used this at work too, there were times when she didn't want to be seen with her eyes closed and a Mona Lisa smile on her face. Instead she practised at home, linking the feelings of being strong, powerful, dynamic and unstoppable to clenching her right fist tightly and saying YES, YES, YES! At work, simply clenching her fist was enough to generate strong positive feelings.

Like many people who start off as rebellious precontemplators, having made the decision to change, Rachel refocused and channelled her energies into mastering the techniques. An unforeseen consequence was her promotion at work to lead the Sales and Negotiation team – her new skills bore unexpected fruit.

SPECIFIC TASKS FOR THIS STAGE

There are other specific tasks that patients must engage in to ensure success in this stage. However well prepared we are on the inside, the outside world has a habit of throwing a banana skin from time to time. There are certain commonsense things patients need to do to avoid slipping, as well as particular areas to focus on.

For those who are smokers, overeaters and drinkers it is mandatory to remove cigarettes, fattening food and alcohol from the home. Failing to do so is asking for trouble. At the first sign of overwhelm it is so easy to engage in the negative habit. Some people like to keep these articles so that they can test their willpower. My advice is always – *don't*. The temptation is always there and I have never seen anyone do this and not succumb at some point. It is not macho bravado, simply foolhardiness.

Likewise it is best to initially avoid the kinds of places that can easily trigger an all-encompassing, overpowering urge. Pubs and clubs are definitely out for starters, as may be fancy restaurants. Offshore workers who can get dirt-cheap cigarettes from 'the bond' are at increased risk of relapse. Drug abusers will definitely need to avoid old friends and old haunts if they are serious in their quest. However, substitute addiction in the form of methadone maintenance seems to be the current professional strategy here.

People can't avoid these negative triggers forever though. At some point they will need to be faced. It is often best to do this as an imaginal role-play first. You can get your patients to rehearse upcoming potentially adverse events in their mind's eye, practising the behaviours they want to use instead. You can augment this further by using the *relaxation response* first, followed by the *enhancing positive emotions* exercise with the particular state that will be most effective in the forthcoming situation. (If you are interested in additional ways to customise this to your patients' needs, with many more examples of specific interventions, consult *Changing with NLP* – see Bibliography.)

Revisit the *three Rs* from Chapter 9. For each key result they want to achieve, your patient will have their motivating reasons together with the specific action steps to which they have committed. Take each action step in turn and use the three additional tactics below to enhance their chances of a successful outcome. The goal of this chapter is to help them put it all into action now and keep the momentum for change heading in the right direction.

Some people like to commit to *written contracts*. These can take various forms. One person may put a sum of money into a personal account for every pound of weight they lose. They can spend this on anything they want for themselves as a reward – as long as it's not food. Others may commit a certain amount of money to charity (though do remember public commitments in Chapter 9). They can also deposit money into their personal account for any positive behaviour they undertake, such as going to the gym. In this way they reward themselves for using healthy behaviour more regularly rather than simply focusing on the elimination of unhealthy behaviour.

Enlisting aid can be very important when changing behaviours. Announcing to family, friends, work colleagues and so on that you are in the process of making a significant change can give much needed support. As well as using public commitment to enhance internal motivation, other people can be invited to help monitor the new behaviour and give encouragement both at times of success and when the going gets tough. A network of backup can improve self-esteem and let you know you're not in it by yourself. Having an exercise partner for example can markedly increase your commitment to show up and get down to work.

Tasking can be used at any stage, though it is often useful here. Agreed tasks can range from doing an 'enhancing positive emotions' exercise every day for a month and reporting back with the results, to keeping a diary of consumption of healthy foods. The task is agreed jointly between you and the patient, needs to be onerous (though not too hard), and commits to focusing on and utilising new behaviours. For someone who is unfit and overweight, a specific task to aim for may be to walk a certain distance every second day, building to a particularly challenging yet reachable goal at the end of a month. Tasks require the exercise of discipline and as such can be extremely effective in helping maintain motivation until new behaviour is second nature.

What gets measured tends to get done. Keeping lists of things to do in your head is less likely to create effective action compared to writing it down on paper and checking in on a regular basis. The following very simple chart can be adapted easily to record and monitor the completion of any commitments, tasks, actions and behaviours day by day. You can note each task or commitment down the left side and tick the corresponding box to record its completion. On the surface it may seem simplistic or even naïve to expect major change to result from this – yet the reverse is often true. Over a period of time it can help engrain new behaviours so that they become automatic.

TABLE 10.1: Tasking

Task	Mon	Tues	Wed	Thurs	Fri	Sat	Sun
1							
2							
3							
4							
5							

Chapter 10 outline summary

Taking action

Taking action is all about marshalling your resources and energies and keeping them pointed for long enough in the right direction until the change you want to make becomes bedded in – and as automatic as the problem used to be.

Changing state

Problem behaviours are often the best way we currently have of changing our state for the better, at least temporarily – we need to find more useful ways to do this effectively

Pattern interrupts

- Short rituals that change our state quickly
- Anything that changes our body posture and gestures will change our internal physiological state (martial arts, dancing, jogging, skipping etc)
- Write down several different ways you can do this for yourself

Changing focus

- Use mental imagery to distance from negative thought processes by shrinking the pictures down, moving them beyond arm's reach, making them black and white
- Enhance positive emotions by reliving powerful memories, making the pictures bigger, brighter, closer with surround sound as you step inside them again

Relaxing rituals

- Trigger the relaxation response by engaging the parasympathetic nervous system
- Allow each out-breath to last twice as long as the in-breath

Specific stage tasks

- Clear the house of temptation (cigarette, food, alcohol etc.)
- Master relaxation skills and enhancing positive emotions
- Revisit the three Rs and make sure they have an action plan
- Commit to a written contract
- Enlist the aid of family, friends, colleagues etc.
- What gets measured gets done . . . fill out a task sheet that they commit to doing

You, me and them

Language conveys multiple perspectives. In any consultation or negotiation there are always – at the very least – three different positions or viewpoints that we can take about the present situation. These are identified by the personal pronouns of first, second and third position language (I, you/we and he/she/it/they). In other words, we need to examine situations from our own standpoint, that of our current communication partner and any other third party interests that may also be concerned or implicated.

For example, as the patient, you and I may be in consultation about an alcohol problem that involves not only you, but also family members, friends, work colleagues and drinking buddies. We may all have differing views and opinions as to whether the issue with alcohol is really a problem at all and certainly what, if anything, needs to be done about it. Failing to examine up front the useful information contained in each of these perspectives will usually lead to a half-hearted solution that works for a bit then fails.

Third person language, when we speak *about* other people who are not here right now, can also be used with inanimate objects. Alcohol itself is often perceived as an 'it', yet it is perniciously imbued with many human characteristics – attraction, power, excitement, confidence etc. It is very easy to project our own dissociated deeper needs onto a third party object to which we then reach out in times of stress or distress as a vehicle for symptomatic relief. The same thing happens of course with cigarettes, drugs, food, shopping, and so on, and before we know it, this 'third party' is actually running our lives. It may seem glib to say, but 're-owning' these projected anthropomorphic qualities is often the key to a lasting solution.

POSITIONS IN PERSPECTIVE

We often see things entirely through our own eyes and the filters of our current beliefs and values from which our behaviours flow. This *first position* perspective allows us to act in each situation from a deep sense of what is important to us, making our needs known, defending our boundaries (physical, emotional, mental) and being 'true' to ourselves. In this position we act with congruence and integrity to get what we want in a cooperative and mutually satisfying way.

Sometimes, however, our truth can hurt. We may come across as overbearing, arrogant, insensitive, disrespectful or worse if we fail to consider – or even dismiss – the beliefs, values, concerns and expectations of others. This is a perspective often met in the stage of 'raising awareness', when reluctant, rebellious, resigned or rationalising precontemplators fail to recognise a developing problem or, worse still, shoot the messenger.

When we step into another person's shoes and try on their perspective of a given situation as if we were them, then we have engaged a *second position* standpoint. If we can, for a moment, drop our preconceived notions and fully appreciate what is happening in this person's world – without judgment or condemnation – then we create a 'we' space (technically first person plural). This is a space of empathy and rapport where we are more in tune with the emotional nuances and feeling states of our communication partner. It can also lead to a more fruitful intellectual understanding of the current situation. This clarity and reciprocated comprehension can in itself be the catalyst of much change.

However, many people can step in and fail to come back out – metaphorically speaking. This is akin to putting someone else's needs ahead of your own. If you do this regularly it is a recipe for stress, burnout, general misery and low self-esteem. This is a fairly typical structure of co-dependency patterns where, in certain contexts, boundaries dissolve and we find ourselves repeating unwanted and destructive behaviours almost against our will. The incongruency thus generated is often a trigger for an escape mechanism – the 'usual suspects' being cigarettes, alcohol, drug of choice etc. We can often recognise this pattern in the stage of 'resolving ambivalence' when people seem to have a co-dependent relationship with their problem, making it difficult to let go and move on to the next stage.

Taking a detached perspective is a bit like stepping back and viewing yourself in a particular situation from a distance – a bit like a fly on the wall. This *third position* dissociated perspective can allow you to re-examine various life experiences with much less emotional charge. You can reflectively think *about* the event rather than being sucked back into any negative feelings associated with it. In this way you can have an opportunity to safely learn something new and update your behaviours accordingly. This is a useful skill to possess and can even be used in the here and now during potentially stressful life events.

Some people, though, may spend much of their lives wandering around in this kind of detached state. They can appear immune both to the stresses and strains and also to the pleasant experiences in life, which may seem to flit ephemerally by. Their air of austerity can make them seem unapproachable – a 'cold fish'. Given that change often requires the right admixture of emotions and intellect they may be found bereft of access to the kinds of feeling states needed to nurture and sustain the change process (motivation, determination, commitment, discipline and so on). In fact they are often the people that others may say 'need' to change, but they are much less likely to present of their own accord.

You can literally 'hear' all three positions in the everyday spoken language of your patient as they describe their presenting problem situation. This can provide useful cues about how they are structuring their experience and what you can do to intervene. Skilfully utilising all three perspectives together can facilitate both a useful understanding of a current problem and simultaneously catalyse an effective solution.

The following process, although usually effective in exploring relationship issues, can actually be used with any problem or symptom whatsoever, often with insightful shifts. Think about a person with whom you have recurrent difficulties. As you remember the last meeting you had with them, cycle through the different perspectives in the exercise below using the diagram to help you sort out each position. It may help to mark them out on the floor on sheets of paper.

Box A The relationship process

1 Step into first position

   Imagine the other person across from you in your mind's eye. Notice how they stand/sit/walk/talk/breathe/move etc. *Look* at their eyes, direction of gaze, tilt of head and whether they are looking towards or away from you. Notice their posture and gestures. *Listen* to their voice. Is it fast/slow/loud/soft/deep/shrill? Which words are emphasised? What are you thinking and feeling in this relationship? What makes it difficult? How do you feel and where in your body do you feel that feeling? Now step out, go neutral and shake it all off!

2 Second position

   Imagine stepping into the shoes of the other person. Try them on for size and fit. Use *their* posture and *their* gestures. Become them as completely as you can. Look across at that 'you' over there in first position. How does that 'you' walk/talk/sit/stand/breathe/move etc.? Go through all the other questions as in step 1 and end by naming the feeling and where you feel it in your body (as them). Now step out, go neutral and shake it all off!

3 Third position

   Step into third position and view the relationship dispassionately from

---

a distance. Who is triggering what in this situation? How do they reinforce one another? Now turn your attention to the first position 'you'. How is he/she coping with the situation? How do 'you' . . . here . . . respond to that 'you' . . . there? What advice would you give that 'you'? What should that 'you' do more of? Less of?

4 Fourth position

Step into a fourth position, *disconnected from the other three.* Allow any residual emotions to go back to the positions where they belong. Think about how the 'third position you' is relating to the 'first position you'. What is the predominant reaction/state/feeling of third position? Now *mentally switch* your first position and third position reactions spatially. Quickly replace one with the other.

5 Return to first position

This time, *take the new way of thinking and feeling* from third position into this, a *revised and updated first position.* Experience the new feelings as you look across at the other person in second position. What has changed now? What is different? How do they look/sound/breathe/move etc. (Revisit the original questions if you wish.) How are you resourceful now? How does this allow you to act differently? Now step out and shake the feelings off.

6 Revisit second position

Step into second position once again, experiencing the 'other' person. See how the 'new you' in first position has changed. Revisit the original questions if you wish. How is the relationship different now?

7 Come home

Return to the updated first position in the here and now and contemplate what will be different in the future.

(Note: you can use a shortened version of the above by simply visiting the first three positions then 'coming home'.)

It is often interesting, if initially somewhat bizarre, to explore the experience of how someone relates to a cigarette, a bottle of whisky, a needle and syringe, various foodstuffs, etc. Using the mental idea of the object as the second position perspective you can get them to associate into that standpoint as they look back at themselves in first position. From here they often get in touch with various disconnected resources (e.g. confidence, inner strength, power, attraction), which have been projected onto the inanimate object. The relationship process allows them to 're-own' these resources and take them back into a first position perspective. From here there is often a dawning realisation that they now have

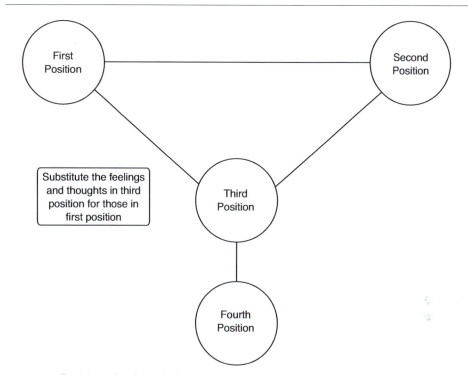

FIGURE B Positions for the relationship process

full access to these states *independent* of the cigarette/bottle/drug etc. This can have a profound effect on future behaviour.

CONSULTING PERSPECTIVES

As a health practitioner you can use various elements of the three perspectives in your everyday consultations. An effective first position allows you to deal congruently and assertively when patients present with challenging issues that push your boundaries. It is not uncommon at times in the addictions field to feel as if you are in some way being manipulated to do something you would prefer not to. Good boundaries will help you when setting useful outcomes for this particular consultation and to maintain professional ethics and behaviours. Although do beware lest too strong a position becomes arrogance. Whilst it is very important to visit the other two positions from time to time, coming back home to a congruent first position is a vital consulting tool.

Sometimes, though, it can be difficult to understand just where another person is coming from. Their presenting issues may seem rather odd or even bizarre. It may be obvious to you and everyone else that they have a problem that may deteriorate into a significant health challenge – but not to them! This is when it is most useful to get a second position perspective. Not only will you gain some insightful clues as to how to proceed next, you will also deepen rapport and give the other person a sense of reassurance that you are attempting to gain some mutual understanding.

For example, when someone has a fixed delusion, trying to argue them out of it is generally futile. However, if you can accept *how* the delusion works to structure their world view you can, by pacing and leading, use the 'logic' of their own internal rules to help them make better behavioural choices. If a person has paranoid ideas it can be useful to tell them to treat with suspicion anything you say because even though it is your intention to be helpful you may inadvertently and unintentionally say or do something that is not helpful. Paradoxically, this statement can make you seem very trustworthy in their eyes because you are using their internal logic in exactly the same way they do.

Many health practitioners are very good at getting rapport – often too good. They step into second position and fail to come out. They live through the emotional roller-coaster narratives of their clients as if they are experiencing it themselves. If you do this with three depressed patients in a row you may feel like you've gone through a wringer. This can be a sure-fire recipe for stress and burnout. In these situations, learning how to take a third person perspective can be highly therapeutic. Reflecting on what has happened as if observing yourself from a distance, dissociating from any overwhelming emotions, can prove a valuable learning experience.

Third position is also a good place to be when handling difficult or aggressive people. Not only does this allow you to reduce your own negative feelings, it helps avoid taking things personally and allows you to focus more on the *process* of the consultation and what needs to happen next. Third position is especially good for planning, particularly when there may be multiple needs to coordinate. It allows for a much wider perspective and exploration of potential consequences of different action plans. Of course, taking the steps to put any plan into action is best done from first position.

This is often the key difference for patients between the stages of preparing to make changes (*see* Chapter 9) and taking action (*see* Chapter 10). If they are still talking *about* the steps they are going to take then you know they are still dissociated to some degree. When they actually take the steps the talk stops – other than to report on progress.

I encourage you to play around with these three perspectives in your consultations. If you video them for reflective learning you can note which position both you and your patients adopt at the various stages. The more facile you become in utilising this important skill the more effective you will be across a range of presenting issues.

Interlude 5 outline summary

Positions in perspective

Language conveys multiple perspectives. Three primary viewpoints are first, second and third position language (*I, you/we and he/she/they/it*)

First position

- See through our own eyes
- Maintain our own boundaries, beliefs, values
- Act congruently to achieve outcomes
- Can sometimes come across as arrogant, overbearing, insensitive

Second position

- Imagine stepping into another person's shoes
- Creates empathy and rapport
- Aids mutual understanding
- Can lead to stress, burnout and co-dependency if overdone

Third position

- A 'fly on the wall' perspective
- A detached, dissociated viewpoint
- A good position for making plans
- Can come across as austere and unapproachable if overdone

The relationship process

- Take a situation involving a difficult or dysfunctional relationship
- Mark out the three positions on the floor
- Visit each space in turn and see through the eyes of that perspective
- Return to your 1st position viewpoint with new, updated information
- Decide what you will do differently in the next 'real-life' encounter

Consulting perspectives

You can use the three positions to enhance your consultation effectiveness
- First – Helps maintain good boundaries in challenging situations
  Beware of owning the 'only right thing to do'
- Second – Helps gain useful information about odd or bizarre presentations
  Beware of becoming 'stuck' in the patient's narrative
- Third – Good for handling difficult/aggressive people
  Beware of becoming overly bureaucratic

CHAPTER 11

Staying on track

It is easy to get lulled into a false sense of security, especially if the 'taking action' stage has gone without any hitches. Complacency can creep in and occasionally an overconfidence that borders on arrogance can surface. It's as if we forget all the effort it has taken to get this far. This is a dangerous time and it is all too easy for a minor lapse to begin the slide down the slippery slope to relapse. Unfortunately, in any single behavioural change attempt, the odds are stacked far more in favour of relapse.

Successfully staying on track demands long-term effort. Stress and overwhelm are often the triggers that cause old behaviours to surface. These occasions are often highly unpredictable. One patient of mine, a regular crash dieter, added up that over the years she had lost 240 lbs in weight. Unfortunately, she also regained 280 lbs. Eating was her major strategy in dealing with stress across all contexts of life.

The immortal words, 'I'll just have the one', often come back to haunt. These are the times when your old problems seem distanced if not forgotten, until they arise unbidden from the swamp, grab you by the throat and pull you back down. Although it is possible, it is very difficult to play around with your old habit as if you are in complete control of picking it up and putting it down again. Most people can't have just one cigarette, one drink or one drug of choice. Yet many people like the excitement of dicing with this danger.

Giving up an old behaviour can sometimes feel just like a bereavement – almost like the loss of an old friend. Some people can find themselves spiralling down into mourning and depression, feeling quite flat and not really engaging with life. It's not altogether surprising. Our problems have had tentacles that reached into many areas of our life. They performed many useful functions, from generating excitement and a reason to live (for some with drug addictions) to giving us feelings of comfort and contentment, however temporary (binge eating). Without adequate replacement, life can seem devoid of pleasure.

Commitment remains an important commodity in staying on track, from which the discipline needed to stay the pace can emerge. In the 'taking action' stage, commitment seems fresh and energising, rising swiftly to get the new tasks started. Over the long haul, though, it must transform into dedication and perseverance that, time and time again, surface during difficult moments (and even hours and perhaps days) to prevent derailment. It pays to have well-ingrained instructions for dire emergencies.

Key to staying on track is to avoid a minor lapse turning into a relapse. For too many people, a relapse is like an on-off light switch. You're either a smoker or a nonsmoker, a drinker or a nondrinker, a normal eater or a binger, there is no in between. Of course this can become a self-fulfilling prophecy of doom and gloom and 'I told you so' recriminations. It is important to prepare people for potential lapses and see this as a normal part of the change process. The unearthing of new information about triggers in a challenging situation allows the opportunity to further fine-tune the change process. In an odd sort of way, lapses can actually help people get the permanent change they desire.

MAINTAINING COMMITMENT

Commitment wanes when people have successfully managed to keep their old behaviours at bay for any length of time and challenges have become fewer and further between. Complacency doesn't bite – it merely snuggles up closely and enticingly. Sometimes commitment wanes because of the 'it's not my fault' syndrome. This generally occurs when people don't take full responsibility for making the change themselves. If it was all due to the brilliant strategies of the clinician – and some clinicians like to foster this myth – or the 'special pill' that cured the ill, then there has been no cultivation of an internal locus of control. When problems arise, as they will invariably do, 'I' can't help it.

In this situation it is vital for the clinician to attribute any success, small or large, to the patient. When you review your patients from time to time it's important to ask questions in a way that not only uncovers 'success stories' but also completes the loop by getting the patient to own the change.

> **Box 11.1 Success story questions**
> What's been different since we last met?
> What's improved most since I last saw you?
> What's the best thing that's happened since our last meeting?
> How did you manage to do that?
> Tell me the part you played in that success?
> Even if you don't know exactly how you caused this to happen . . . guess!

Commitment also wanes when people forget just how bad it used to be. At these times it can be helpful to dig out the decision balance sheet from the 'resolving ambivalence' stage. Look again particularly at what it will cost them if they return to the old behaviours. Get them to think of what they've currently got that they might lose. Imagine what that loss might prevent them from doing in the future. Remember that people will often do far more to prevent a loss than they will to make a gain.

Ask your patients:

What will it cost you if you give up now?

What will you stand to lose?

For both you and them, write out a new list and keep it handy (in a wallet or purse) for when either temptation bites or overwhelm looms unexpectedly large and breathes down your neck. In these situations looking at the list can provide the impetus for remaining on track. They can print out their list from a computer, write it on a special card in a particular colour of ink and personalise it in any way that makes it more meaningful for them. Get them to commit to referring to it at the first signs of a downward slip and any other time they feel themselves wavering on the brink.

Box 11.2 What it will cost me if I give up now?

1

2

3

4

5

6

7

8

9

10

DIRE EMERGENCY

Note to reader: this section is written as 'you' rather than 'them' to directly personalise the 'dire emergency' message.

When things get really tough and you feel the rug beginning to be pulled out from under your feet, you are entering a state of dire emergency. You will have your own internal equivalent of flashing blue lights and sirens. You are likely to be in a negative state and in danger of being dragged down into the mire from which the only escape may appear to be your old behaviour. These are difficult times and you must take action quickly.

The main priority is to change your state as rapidly as possible. Remember that physical action is the swiftest way to change how you feel. You already have a list of *instant state changers* (*see* Chapter 10) and it is time to put these into action. Make sure that you know which of the actions on your list will reliably and effectively do the job. Don't think – just *do it*. If you are in a situation involving other people then you *must* excuse yourself immediately and go for a time out. Do whatever it takes to diminish the negative feelings.

As the negative feelings subside you can remember why you are making this change in the first place. You can recite the benefits over and over in your mind's ear. Then summon up your positive imagery of resourceful times, events and feelings and feel it wrap around you like a comfort blanket. At this point you may choose to contact a friend for further support until your internal world stabilises.

Write out the following on a card and keep it handy.

Box 11.3 Dire emergency card

1 Use an instant state changer
2 Go for a time out
3 Recite the benefits of changing
4 Summon positive imagery
5 Phone a friend

LAPSE AND RELAPSE

A lapse is when you have a slip and briefly revert to the problem behaviour. A relapse is when you completely revert to your old ways, as if the change never occurred. You can really only have a lapse or a relapse if you have already succeeded in making a change. In effect they are actually both signs of achievement. People who haven't started the change process can have neither. You can only lose something that you have previously attained. This may seem a strange reframe as most consider relapsing to mean that they have failed, or worse still, that *they* are a failure – confusing behaviour with identity. However, the real failure is if you never take a step on the path towards getting what you really want.

Some people rely upon 'magical' thinking when they start to make changes. They believe it should all go very smoothly from start to finish. If it doesn't it means they didn't think and project the right kinds of thoughts to make the rest of the world play its part in realising their inner fantasies. This is like trying to control the uncontrollable. However good the plan, however strong the resolve, there will always be potential setbacks on the path to lasting change. Some are predictable, others entirely unexpected.

When unlooked-for problems arise it is easy for the wind to be taken out of your sails. Often, the all-or-nothing thinking that prevails in these moments turns what could be seen as a minor blip into an overwhelmingly huge, out-of-proportion disaster that totally engulfs you – and before you know it, you have completely relapsed. It can seem as if all your hard work was for nothing. This kind of 'on-off' binary thinking, where you are totally one thing or the other (smoker/nonsmoker, drinker/nondrinker etc.) is very dangerous.

Given that lapses are an invariable hazard on the path to change, it seems rather silly if we bury our heads in the sand and ignore their potential occurrence. And that is exactly what some patients do – sometimes even ably assisted by their clinicians. It is as if by contemplating it out in the open then we will, by magical thinking, cause the lapse to occur. Best to pretend it won't crop up.

In fact the reverse is actually more likely to happen. By actively seeking out times, places and events where lapse can occur, we can plan to forestall it by adequate preparation. However – and this is very important – by actually rehearsing a lapse happening and seeing yourself get up, dust yourself down, learn the lesson and get back with the programme, you are installing a vital recovery strategy to help you stay on track. Prescribing a lapse can be a vital tactic to increase your overall chances of successful change. Think of the particular problem behaviour you indulged in as you read through the following exercise.

Box 11.4 Prescribing a lapse

Sit down, make yourself comfortable and breathe easily.
In your mind's eye, imagine everything is going very smoothly for a week or two – enjoy the feeling.
Now see yourself having an unexpected difficulty.
Imagine that, despite yourself, you indulge in your problem behaviour.
Notice all the consequences that ensue – and how bad it feels.
Now see yourself strengthening your resolve as you recommit to taking the necessary action to immediately get back on track.
Picture how you stand, walk, talk, breathe as you rededicate yourself.
Notice the lessons you have learned from this encounter.
How does this help you to deal more effectively with these situations should they arise again?

As a clinician, prescribing a lapse, although it can seem counterintuitive, is a strategy that has interesting results. Firstly it takes the heat off your patient and avoids the anxiety generated by the need to do things perfectly first time. This can afford much relief. It also acknowledges that real life rarely runs smoothly without some form of challenge and potential setback. Paradoxically, by suggesting a lapse is likely to occur you are actually decreasing the chances of its occurrence. Even if it does happen, you have already installed a recovery strategy, which by rehearsal will ensure that rather than a downward spiral to full relapse, the lapse is merely a stumble on the path. Prescribing a lapse can result in a 'win-win' solution.

This exercise also gives an opportunity once again to predict difficult times ahead and prepare in advance. It can then be very useful to identify the very skills, attitudes, signature strengths and resources that your patient can bring to bear in those challenging situations. Further imaginal rehearsal with these firmly in place beforehand will afford even more flexibility of response when they arise (*see* Putting strengths to work, pages 116–17).

RHONA'S LAPSE

Rhona went through the visual imagery lapse exercise, saw herself bingeing after a week of doing well, feeling the immediate pangs of regret then summoning the strength to get back on track again. It was just as well she did. Nearly two weeks after congratulating herself on how well she was doing in real life, she came face to face with her first lapse.

She saw her ex-partner in town with his 'new woman'. Although it had been three years since their split she felt the anguish and pain of rejection all over again. That evening the feelings of being alone and unloved welled up and, unable to console herself, she turned once again to the one thing that she knew would give her at least temporary relief – food.

Afterwards she felt sick, guilty and full of remorse at her actions. However, rather than lapsing into a customary downward spiral, she felt the initial stirrings of a new feeling – an inner strength which although it began as a flicker, rose to become a calm 'centredness', like being in the eye of a storm. She replayed the memory of the encounter with her ex-partner earlier in the day. This time she felt as if she was a still, quiet, composed observer of the event, rather than a piece of flotsam tossed in a stormy sea.

Afterwards she had the strange feeling that she was seeing the whole of their relationship, from beginning to end, in a new light. She vowed that she would never again allow any man to make her feel that way. If they couldn't accept her as she was, that was their loss. This decision was a major catalyst in fostering her increasing self-acceptance.

WHEN RELAPSE OCCURS

No matter how badly we want things to be different, and despite our best efforts at the time, for some people relapse is part of the change process. It can occur days, weeks, months and even years after the original change took place. Just when we thought it was safe, disaster strikes. It often catches us completely by surprise and we may be caught up in intense feelings of disappointment and frustration.

There are many reasons for relapsing. The commonest is some form of overwhelming stress or distress that leaves us bereft of coping skills. We are swamped, feel as if we are sinking and reach out for the one thing that helped us cope in the past – whether that is a cigarette, a drink or food. Sally who had stopped binge eating three years previously found herself in a situation of being bullied at work. Caught in the tension between wanting to confront it, yet feeling small, overpowered and helpless, she started bingeing again.

Intense emotions such as anger, fear or depression often leave us rudderless. Whilst we may be able to avoid social situations or people who push our buttons, it is far more difficult to avoid our own inner thoughts and feelings. Wherever we go, there we are. We cannot escape from ourselves that easily. Too few of us have learnt to deal effectively in healthy ways with these negative emotions. Chapter 9 shows you some useful strategies that can prepare you to handle these states more successfully and insulate you from distress.

Other people are a big factor in relapse, especially if they engage in the same problem behaviour. They can bring a great deal of pressure to bear to get you to revert to your old behaviours. Your change process may threaten them. They may not like the new you or may find your new ways of being in the world intimidating. To restore their own status quo they may urge you to 'just have the one . . . it won't hurt you'. If you have stopped meeting up with friends because the socialising takes place in a challenging situation for you (e.g. the pub), then you may feel quite lonely. The hankering for reconnection is a double-edged sword. The price of friendship may be your sobriety.

Some people try to push themselves through change by sheer willpower. They don't avail themselves of the many diverse techniques that can aid them. Perhaps they use the wrong change process at the wrong time, or they keep on with the same strategy that has consistently failed them in the past. This can lead to intense frustration, with almost inevitable consequences.

Too many smokers find themselves putting on weight as they try to satisfy the 'hand-mouth' reflex. They substitute one problem behaviour for another. For some people, the underlying problem is actually an eating issue. They have used smoking as a means of weight control. It is useful to keep this in mind for the next attempt at stopping so you can ensure they have other choices available.

Lessons to learn

Relapse affects people differently. Some do seem to go all the way back to the beginning, as if they'd never changed at all. They may become demoralised, defeated and dejected. In this kind of state they may remain defensive and ignore your efforts at further help.

Most of the others, however, cycle back a stage or two in the change process, regroup and try again. Relapse is often a time of inner conflict when you become aware that a certain trigger or situation has changed the direction you wanted to go in. This is an important learning point as it harbours the seeds of successful future change.

In essence the conflict is a form of ambivalence and can be resolved by means of the various approaches in Chapter 8. You can unearth some previously hidden benefits of the problem behaviour and utilise this in further fine-tuning the next attempt. Looked at this way, the relapse has thrown up some very useful information that will further strengthen the change when it occurs.

For others the relapse may only be as far as the 'preparing to make changes' stage. Rather than being defeated they are already planning what they can do differently next time and are galvanising their energies for the attempt. This may involve not only learning the lesson of the relapse but also deciding if a different approach or technique may pay higher dividends this time. Focusing on generating commitment to renewed action is a key launch pad to success.

Here are some vital questions to ask anyone who has had a relapse.

Box 11.5 Learning from relapse

What was the specific trigger that caused the relapse?
What skill did you need instead in this situation?
What hidden positives have you unearthed?
What is the most important thing you have learned about yourself from this situation?
How will you deal with this situation differently next time?
What will you do instead . . . what steps will you take?
What other skills, resources and attitudes would help you?
Are there any other complications you need to prepare for?
What is the smallest next step you can take right now?

Once you have identified not only the stumbling blocks that led to the relapse but also the lessons that these experiences afford us, it is vital that you incorporate this newfound knowledge into your ensuing action plan. You may want to respecify the three Rs to include any new results, reasons and right actions you want to take. Rededicating yourself to the task in hand requires renewal of commitment. You will also want to do an imaginal rehearsal, seeing yourself employing the necessary skills in the kinds of contexts that triggered the relapse – this time with a successful outcome. Keep honing your imagery and adding any other resources that will get you back on track. Remember to make the next attempt at changing an inevitability – plan for *when* it will occur rather than *if*.

Life, then, always presents us with many opportunities for relapse. It can be an inescapable component of the change process and one that, despite our best plans, may sneak up on us unawares. In truth, lasting change demands that we effectively negotiate these potential obstacles time and time again. We must do so in a way that resolves the inherent conflicts they throw up, allowing a deeper integration of our fledgling new behaviours until they become an automatic and robust part of our daily life.

ROBERT'S RELAPSE

Binge drinking is not usually solved in a 'one step and you're free' scenario. Sadly this proved to be the case for Robert. Despite the motivation that came from the shame of his drink-driving offence, he found maintaining sobriety a struggle. He missed the socialising with his mates down the pub and became increasingly irritable with his wife and family. He had no major hobbies or interests and spent more time ensconced in front of the television flicking aimlessly between sports channels.

After a month, Robert's mates took his fate into their own hands. If Robert wasn't going to go to the pub then the pub would come to Robert. One evening they turned up on his doorstep with a crate of beer. The rest, as they say, is history. Robert started going back to the pub 'just to be sociable'. However, being sociable soon led to the inevitable return to old ways. To a large extent, it was as if he had never been away.

Robert's relapse continued for the best part of six months. It was only with his court case looming large on the horizon (it had been delayed several times already) that he once again turned his thoughts to what to do about his drinking. He knew that, in the long term, abstinence was the only real solution. He just didn't know if he had the energy to sustain that kind of commitment.

He felt very conflicted about the thought of having to 'give up' his mates at the pub. He really couldn't see himself sitting sipping a glass of orange whilst they all imbibed. On the one hand stood friendship, socialisation and drinking whilst on the other was sobriety, loneliness and time weighing heavily on his hands. He recognised at an intellectual level the benefits to his overall health and well-being that sobriety would bring. However, he wasn't yet sure enough in his gut that he could make the pledge. All in all it felt to him very much like a bereavement – he seemed damned whatever he option he chose.

In consultation, he gained some clarity on how he was motivated to move away from the pain his habit caused but had not yet devised life-sustaining strategies that could pull him in a positive direction. He recognised that friendship and socialisation were important to him but up until now he had no access to other avenues that fulfilled these needs. He also saw that he would need to replace aimless nights in front of the television with doing something more productive.

Fate lent a hand in a positive way. Whilst he had never seen himself as an alcoholic and would in no way be tempted to go to Alcoholics Anonymous, he bumped into a former heavy-drinking friend who had successfully gone down that route. Mick, sober for five years, was now an avid bowls player. He invited Robert to come along and give it a try. Initially he felt his old feelings of insecurity and lack of confidence begin to rise up. However, he determined to give it a go and see what happened. After all, he could always back out if he felt too uncomfortable.

To his surprise he found that the bowls club had a wide range of ages in its membership. He had thought they would all be much older than him – they weren't. Not only that, they were friendly and welcoming as well as being at times fiercely competitive when 'on the green'. He quickly found himself as the third man in a team of four and before long was inveigled into the local league. With both indoor and outdoor seasons he realised that this was a year-round activity which he could enjoy. Very soon he was playing two or three times a week.

As well as taking up bowls, Robert also looked for an activity that could keep him busy at home. Way back in his youth he had developed an interest in wood carving and building small models. He bought himself a few bits and pieces and got started again. One of his tricks had been to make 'ships in a bottle'. These were replicas of sailing ships that seemed impossibly tall-masted to fit into the neck of a small bottle – unless you knew the secret. Once he had produced a few he found that several of his bowls colleagues wanted one and orders for more came in.

Slowly but surely, Robert found that his new interests not only gave him the friendship and status that his drinking used to, but also that he became slimmer and felt fitter and more clear-headed as a result. He knew that his battles with alcohol were not over but he recognised his increasing resolve to tackle any potential difficulties head-on rather than reach for the bottle.

Chapter 11 outline summary

Staying on track
Lapses and relapses are a normal part of the change process
Key to staying on track is preventing a minor lapse becoming a major relapse

Maintaining commitment
Over the long haul, commitment evolves into dedication and perseverance
- Ask 'success story' questions to maintain an internal locus of control
- What will it cost you if you give up now?
- What will you stand to lose?
- Write out a personalised list

Dire emergency card
It is useful to have a card written with specific instructions about what to do in times of difficulty
- When the going gets tough remember to use instant state changers
- Remove yourself from the situation if possible
- Re-establish positive emotions and imagery
- Reconnect to your skills and resources

Lapse and relapse
- *Lapse* – you have a slip and briefly revert to the problem behaviour
- *Relapse* – you completely revert to old habits
You can only have a lapse/relapse if you have already succeeded in making a change

Prescribing a lapse
- Lapses are an invariable hazard in the process of change
- We need to prepare for their occurrence
- Installing a recovery strategy prevents lapse becoming relapse
- Paradoxically, prescribing a lapse may reduce the chances of its occurrence

When relapse occurs
- It can occur days, weeks, months and even years after the original change took place
- Common reasons are stress, distress and overwhelm
- Intense negative emotions are often a factor

- Other people with the same problem can exert negative pressure
- Willpower is not a substitute for using effective strategies
- Substitute behaviours may cause their own problems (e.g. weight gain on stopping smoking)

Learning from relapse
- Relapse affects people differently
- Identify which stage of the change process they have cycled back to
- Resolve the incongruencies and ambivalences that have arisen
- Ask the 'learning from relapse' questions
- Incorporate this knowledge into a new action plan for change

Modal operators

These are words that convey both possibility and necessity together with their negative counterparts. Between these poles lie differing degrees of probability of something happening (i.e. a behavioural shift). As you become skilled you will find yourself weaving sentences artfully to enable a patient to move from a stuck pattern, from which change appears unlikely, to being open to the possibility of creating a different future altogether – and then take action.

You can practise by choosing words from each section then constructing sentences which flow from one to the other seamlessly. Start simply with two types then build to as many as six or more (*see* page 28).

TABLE 1A Modal operators

NEGATIVE NECESSITY	NECESSITY
Doesn't allow	Allow
Don't have to	Have to
Mustn't	Must
Ought not	Ought
Shouldn't	Should
Not supposed to	Supposed to
IMPROBABILITY	**PROBABILITY**
Couldn't	Could
May not	May
Might not	Might
Wouldn't	Would
Don't let	Let
Had better not	Had better
IMPOSSIBILITY	**POSSIBILITY**
Am not	Able to
Can't	Can
Don't choose to	Choose to
Won't	Will
Impossible	Possible
Doesn't permit	Permits

Bibliography

Botelho, Rick. *Motivational Practice: promoting healthy habits and self-care of chronic disease.* New York: MHH Publications; 2002.

Feldman, Mitchell D and Christensen, John F, editors. *Behavioral Medicine in Primary Care.* 2nd ed. New York: Lange Medical Books/McGraw Hill; 2003.

Duncan, Barry L, Miller, Scott D and Sparks, Jacqueline A. *The Heroic Client: a revolutionary way to improve effectiveness through client directed, outcome informed therapy.* San Francisco: Jossey-Bass Inc; 2000.

Hubble, Mark A, Duncan, Barry L and Miller, Scott D, editors. *The Heart and Soul of Change: what works in therapy.* Washington DC: American Psychological Association; 1999.

Loehr, Jim and Schwartz, Tony. *On Form.* London: Nicholas Brealey Publishing; 2003.

Miller, William R and Rollnick, Stephen. *Motivational Interviewing: preparing people for change.* 2nd ed. New York: The Guilford Press; 2002.

Prochaska, James O, Norcross, John C and DiClemente, Carlo C. *Changing for Good.* New York: Harper Collins; 1994.

Rollnick, Stephen, Mason, Pip and Butler, Chris. *Health Behavior Change.* New York: Churchill Livingstone; 1999.

Seligman, Martin. *Authentic Happiness.* London: Nicholas Brealey Publishing; 2003.

Snyder, CR and Lopez, SJ, editors. *Handbook of Positive Psychology.* New York: Oxford University Press; 2002.

Walker, Lewis. *Changing with NLP: a casebook of neuro-linguistic programming in medical practice.* Oxford: Radcliffe Medical Press; 2004.

Walker, Lewis. *Consulting with NLP: neuro-linguistic programming in the medical consultation.* Oxford: Radcliffe Medical Press; 2002.

Index